The 12-Lead ECG in ST Elevation Myocardial Infarction

A PRACTICAL APPROACH
FOR CLINICIANS

T0261411

The 12-Lead ECG in ST Elevation Myocardial Infarction

A PRACTICAL APPROACH FOR CLINICIANS

A. Bayés de Luna, MD, FESC, FACC

Professor of Medicine, Universidad Autonoma Barcelona
Director of Institut Catala de Cardiologia
Hospital Santa Creu i Sant Pau
St. Antoni M. Claret 167
ES-08025
Barcelona
Spain

M. Fiol-Sala, MD

Chief of the Intensive Coronary Care Unit
Intensive Coronary Care Unit
Hospital Son Dureta
Palma
Mallorca
Spain

E. M. Antman, MD

Senior Investigator, TIMI Study Group
Professor of Medicine, Harvard Medical School; *and*
Director of the Samuel A. Levine Cardiac Unit at the Brigham & Women's Hospital
Cardiovascular Division
Brigham and Women's Hospital
75 Francis Street
Boston
USA

With the collaboration of A. Carrillo, J. Cino, I. Cygankiewicz

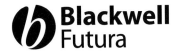

© 2007 Antonio Bayés de Luna, Miguel Fiol-Sala and Elliott Antman
Published by Blackwell Publishing
Blackwell Futura is an imprint of Blackwell Publishing

Blackwell Publishing, Inc., 350 Main Street, Malden, Massachusetts 02148-5020, USA
Blackwell Publishing Ltd, 9600 Garsington Road, Oxford OX4 2DQ, UK
Blackwell Science Asia Pty Ltd, 550 Swanston Street, Carlton, Victoria 3053, Australia

All rights reserved. No part of this publication may be reproduced in any form or by any
electronic or mechanical means, including information storage and retrieval systems, without
permission in writing from the publisher, except by a reviewer who may quote brief passages
in a review.

First published 2007

1   2007

ISBN-13: 978-1-4051-5786-5
ISBN-10: 1-4051-5786-0

Library of Congress Cataloging-in-Publication Data

Bayés de Luna, Antonio.
    The 12 lead ECG in ST elevation myocardial infarction : a practical approach for clinicians /
A. Bayés de Luna, M. Fiol-Sala, E.M. Antman ; with the collaboration of J. Carrillo, J. Cino.,
I. Cygankiewicz.
        p. ; cm.
    Includes bibliographical references and index.
    ISBN-13: 978-1-4051-5786-5
    ISBN-10: 1-4051-5786-0
    1. Myocardial infarction–Diagnosis.   2. Electrocardiography.   I. Bayes de Luna, A. (Antoni)
Fiol-Sala, M. (Miguel)   II. Antman, E. M. (Elliott)   III. Title.   IV. Title: Twelve lead ECG in ST
elevation myocardial infarction.
    [DNLM: 1. Electrocardiography–methods–Programmed Instruction.   2. Myocardial
Infarction–diagnosis–Programmed Instruction. WG 18.2 Z999 2006]

    RC685.I6B37   2006
    616.1′23707547—dc22

                                                                                            2006010108

A catalogue record for this title is available from the British Library

Acquisitions: Gina Almond
Development: Fiona Pattison
Set in 9.5/12 Palatino by TechBooks, India
Printed and bound in India by Replika Press Pvt., Ltd

For further information on Blackwell Publishing, visit our website:
www.blackwellfutura.com

The publisher's policy is to use permanent paper from mills that operate a sustainable forestry
policy, and which has been manufactured from pulp processed using acid-free and elementary
chlorine-free practices. Furthermore, the publisher ensures that the text paper and cover board
used have met acceptable environmental accreditation standards.

Blackwell Publishing makes no representation, express or implied, that the drug dosages in this
book are correct. Readers must therefore always check that any product mentioned in this
publication is used in accordance with the prescribing information prepared by the
manufacturers. The author and the publishers do not accept responsibility or legal liability for
any errors in the text or for the misuse or misapplication of material in this book.

Contents

Foreword

The electrocardiogram (ECG), introduced more than 100 years ago by Einthoven, continues to be a vital clinical resource with constantly evolving new diagnostic and prognostic features. It remains one of the milestones of "bedside diagnosis" as identified more than 50 years ago by the school of Paul Wood. The ECG is the "gold standard" technique for diagnosis of cardiac arrhythmias, conduction disturbances, preexcitation, acute coronary syndromes, and chronic myocardial infarction with Q waves. Furthermore, it is also useful for diagnosis of other heart diseases and a range of different clinical situations because of its simplicity and low cost. Also, there is a good correlation between ECG morphologies, prognosis and some certain types of genetic mutations in channelopathies like long QT syndrome.

The role of ECG in acute coronary syndromes (ACS) is pivotal in patients both with and without ST elevation. The classification of ACS based on the presence or absence of ST elevation on the ECG is very useful to determine which patients need urgent reperfusion. However, beyond this classification, the physician caring for a patient with ST elevation myocardial infarction (STEMI) may obtain by careful observation of ST deviations other meaningful information about the location of the culprit artery, site of occlusion, coronary dominance, and the size of the myocardial area at risk.

The conjunction of skillfulness and expertise in electrocardiography and in coronary care of Antoni Bayes de Luna, Miquel Fiol and Elliott Antman has resulted in the publication of this excellent book, that contains in 100 pages all the current information on the role of the surface ECG in the diagnosis and management of STEMI. The authors, using the concept of the injury vector, perform a double deductive original approach. First, starting from the site of the occlusion, it is explained with clear drawings and ECG coronary angiographic correlations, how the different ECG patterns appear. And second, most important for the physician managing a patient with a STEMI, they discuss how after reviewing the ST deviations in a sequential manner it becomes possible to deduce the culprit artery and the site of occlusion. Furthermore, the book contains other important prognostic clues obtained from the surface ECG. There is also a very well presented self-assessment section.

I believe this book will be extremely useful for all personnel caring for patients with acute coronary syndromes. The application of the information that is contained is quite important in urgent decision-making and in overall management. Furthermore, I strongly recommend this book, not only for all the personnel involved in acute coronary care but, because of its didactic approach, to any clinician wishing to understand how a myocardial infarction evolves and impacts the most important and readily available diagnostic tool: the electrocardiogram.

I congratulate the authors for their vision, and also Blackwell Publishing for the excellence of this work.

Valentin Fuster
Executive Director, Mount Sinai Heart
President, World Heart Federation
Past President, American Heart Association.

Introduction

The scalar ECG is an important diagnostic tool for patients with heart disease and other conditions. Its value is particularly evident in patients with an acute coronary syndrome (ACS) and narrow QRS. It is beyond the scope of this book to discuss the cases of ACS that present with a wide QRS because it is known that these already carry a poor prognosis. The ECG in the cases of narrow QRS is crucial not only for diagnosis but also for prognosis and risk stratification. The ECG is at the center of the decision pathway dividing patients with ACS who show ST elevation (ST elevation myocardial infarction – STEMI) and those without ST elevation (UA/NSTEMI). This distinction is important because of the time urgency of reperfusion in patients with STEMI.

This book offers to cardiologists, specialists in intensive care, physicians working in emergency medicine, interventional cardiologists, and general practitioners insights into the ECG that permit a correct diagnosis and help frame management of STEMI. We explain how for all types of STEMI, the proper use of the concept of the injury vector and knowledge of its direction and its projection in the frontal and horizontal planes, yield a correct interpretation of the deviation of the ST-segment and its correlation with the site of the occlusion, and the area of left ventricle at risk. For each site of coronary occlusion we use a consistent sequence to explain the ECG abnormalities. In a four-part panel we show a schematic of the coronary tree illustrating the point of occlusion (a), the area at risk according to the segmentation of the left ventricle proposed by the North American Societies of Imaging (b), the location of the 17 left ventricular segments in a polar map (c), and the projection of the injury vector on the positive and negative hemifields of the 12-lead scalar ECG.

We appreciate the contribution of Dr. Valentin Fuster who wrote the Foreword for this book, and the efficient staff at Blackwell Publishing who made its publication possible.

CHAPTER 1

The heart walls and coronary circulation

The heart is located in the central-left part of the thorax (lying on the diaphragm) and is oriented anteriorly, with the apex directed forward, downward, and leftward. The myocardium and specific conduction system are perfused by the right coronary artery (RCA), the left anterior descending coronary artery (LAD), and the left circumflex coronary artery (LCX) (Figure 1).

The heart walls and their segmentation: the importance to uniform nomenclature

The left ventricle is cone shaped. Although the limits are imprecise it can be divided, except at the apex, into four walls, named classically septal, anterior, lateral, and inferoposterior (Figure 2).

The basal part of the inferoposterior wall often branches upward and then becomes really posterior and for that reason it was named the posterior wall.

For more than 60 years, the terms posterior infarction, injury, and ischemia have been applied when it was considered that the basal part of the inferoposterior wall was affected (Bayés de Luna 1999, Chou Te-Chuan et al. 1977, Goldman 1964, Kennedy et al. 1970, Wagner 2002).

Other names have been given to the walls of the heart (Roberts & Gardin 1978), but the consensus of the North American Societies of Imaging (Cerqueira 2002) divided the left ventricle into 17 segments and 4 walls – septal, anterior, lateral, and inferior (Figures 3 and 4). This consensus states that the classical inferoposterior wall should be called inferior "for consistency" and segment 4 inferobasal instead of posterior. Figures 3 and 4 show the 17 segments into which the four cardiac walls are divided (6 basal, 6 medial, 4 inferior, and the apex), and in the right side of Figure 4 the heart walls with their corresponding segments on a polar "bull's-eye" map are shown. We believe that this terminology is the most appropriate and facilitates interpretation of the ECG.

If one considers that the heart is located in the thorax strictly in a posteroanterior position, as is presented in a bull's-eye polar map or in transverse images by cardiovascular magnetic resonance (CMR) in the case of involvement (injury or necrosis) of the basal part of the inferior wall (classically called posterior wall), the necrosis vector in a sagittal view would be directed strictly posteroanteriorly. This would produce an RS (R) morphology in V_{1-2} and the injury vector

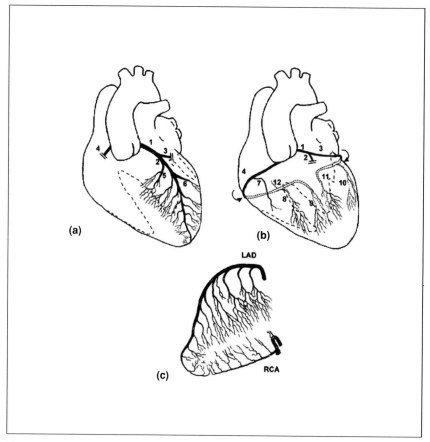

Figure 1 Coronary circulation: (a) territory of the LAD; (b) territory of the RCA and the LCX; (c) septal perfusion. The anterior part is perfused by the septal branches of the LAD and the inferior part by the septal branches of the posterior descending coronary artery (RCA or, less frequently, LCX). Numbers refer to the following elements: (1) left main trunk; (2) LAD; (3) LCX; (4) RCA; (5) first septal branch (S_1); (6) first diagonal branch (D_1); (7) RV branch; (8) posterior descending from the RCA; (9) posterolateral from the RCA; (10) obtuse marginal (OM) from the LCX; (11) posterobasal from the LCX; (12) AV node branch (RCA).

would be registered as ST-segment depression in the same leads (Figure 5a). However, magnetic resonance imaging (Blackwell et al. 1993, Pons-Lladó & Carreras 2005) provides evidence in vivo that in the sagittal view the heart is oriented with an oblique right-to-left inclination and not in a strictly posteroanterior position (Figure 6). This explains why the RS (R)–ST depression pattern in V_1 is a consequence of necrosis injury of the lateral wall (Figure 5c) and that the involvement of the classically named posterior wall (actually the inferobasal segment of the inferior wall) produces ST depression more evident in V_{2-3} than in V_1, and an RS morphology in V_1 (Figure 5b). Other reasons to

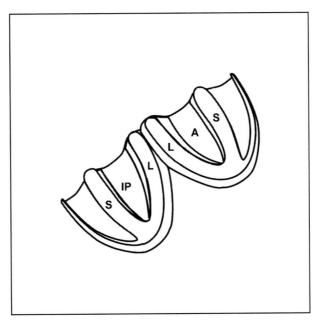

Figure 2 The left ventricle may be divided into four walls that are named anterior (A), inferoposterior (IP), septal (S), and lateral (L). The inferobasal portion of the inferoposterior wall is usually considered the posterior wall.

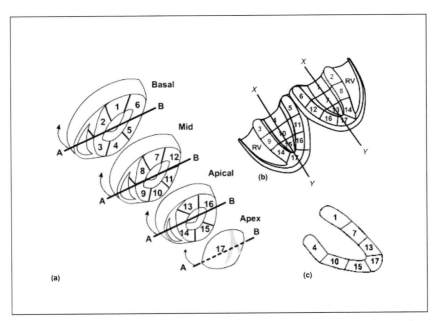

Figure 3 (a) Segments into which the left ventricle is divided according to the transverse sections performed at the basal (B), medial (M), and apical (A) levels (Figure 6). The basal and medial sections delineate six segments each, while the apical section shows four segments. Together with the apex, they constitute the 17 segments into which the left ventricle can be divided, according to the classification performed by the American Imaging Societies (Cerqueira 2002). View of the 17 segments with the heart open in a longitudinal horizontal plane (b) and longitudinal vertical (sagittal-like) plane (c).

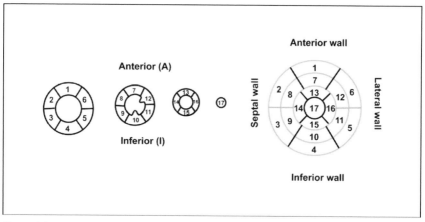

Figure 4 Images of the segments in which the left ventricle is divided according to the cross sections at the basal, medial, and apical levels, considering that the heart is located in the thorax strictly in a posteroanterior position. Segment 4 (inferobasal) was classically named the posterior wall. The basal and medial sections delineate six segments each, while the apical section shows four segments. Note in the middle section the location of the papillary muscles. To the right are all 17 segments in the form of a polar map ("bull's-eye"), just as it is represented in isotopic images.

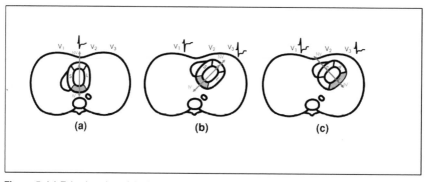

Figure 5 (a) False location of the heart in the thorax. This results from the extrapolation of the classical concepts expressed in the majority of ECG books and the images used by the imaging specialists (Figure 4). According to that, the injury vector (IV) and necrosis vector (NV) that present approximately in the same direction, but in opposite directions, would explain the RS morphology with ST-segment depression observed in V_1 in the case of STEMI, mainly affecting the inferobasal segment (classically posterior wall). However, according to the true heart position in the thorax (b and c), the RS morphology with the largest ST depression in V_1 is explained mainly by the involvement of the lateral wall. (c) When the inferobasal segment is involved, the morphology in V_1 is RS, with smaller ST depression in V_1 than in V_3 because in this case the IV and NV point toward V_3 and not V_1 (b).

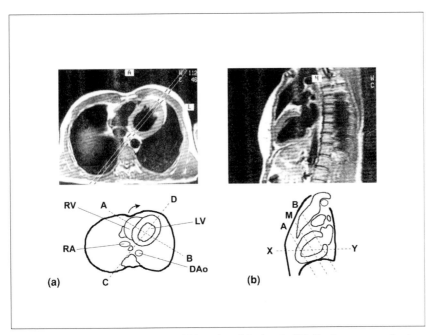

Figure 6 Magnetic resonance imaging. (a) Location of the heart within the thorax, according to a section in the thoracic axial plane (at the level of the line "XY" of b). (b) Note that this longitudinal vertical section presents an oblique direction from backward to forward and from the right to the left (sagittal like) (see line CD in part a) and therefore corresponds with Figure 5b and c and not with Figure 5a.

eliminate use of the word *posterior* are as follows:

1 The posterior wall often does not truly exist because all of the inferoposterior wall lays flat on the diaphragm.

2 Even when necrosis exists, it usually does not generate an R in V_1 (Q equivalent) because the inferobasal segment of the inferior wall depolarizes after 40–50 milliseconds.

Coronary circulation: the perfusion of the heart walls

In Figure 7b–d, the perfusion that the different walls with each of their corresponding segments receive from the three coronary arteries can be seen. The areas with common perfusion are colored in gray in Figure 7a. In Figure 7e the relation between the 12 leads of the surface ECG and the four walls of the heart is shown.

Left anterior descending coronary artery

The LAD perfuses the anterior wall especially via the diagonal branches (segments 1, 7, and 13), the anterior part of the septum via the septal branches (segments 2, 8, and part of 14; segment 14 is sometimes coperfused by the

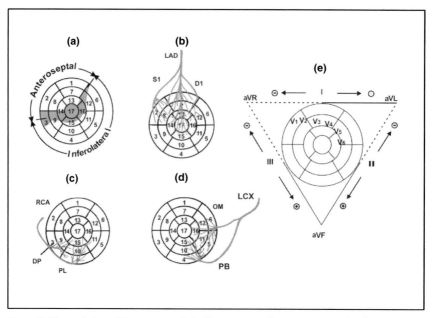

Figure 7 The perfusion of these segments by the corresponding coronary arteries (b to d) can be seen in the "bull's-eye" images. According to the anatomical variants of coronary circulation, there are areas of shared variable perfusion (a). The apex (segment 17) is generally perfused by the LAD, but sometimes by the RCA or even the LCX. Segments 4, 10, and 15 are perfused by the RCA or the LCX, depending on which of them is dominant (the RCA in more than 85% of the cases). Segment 15 is often partially perfused from LAD. (e) Location of the 12-lead ECG in relation to the polar map. Abbreviations: D_1, first diagonal branch; LAD, left anterior descending coronary artery; LCX, left circumflex coronary artery; OM, obtuse marginal branch; PB, posterobasal branch; PD, posterior descending coronary artery; PL, posterolateral branch; RCA, right coronary artery; S_1, first septal branch.

RCA), and often part of segments 3 and 9 that are also shared with the RCA. Frequently, the LAD perfuses the apex and part of the inferior wall, as the LAD wraps around the apex in over 80% of cases (segment 17 and part of segment 15). Also the right bundle branch is perfused by the first septal branch.

Right coronary artery

This artery perfuses, in addition to the right ventricle, the inferior region of the septum (part of segments 3 and 9). Segment 14 corresponds more to the LAD, but is sometimes shared by both arteries. The RCA also perfuses a large part of the inferior wall (segments 4, 10 and 15). Segments 4 and 10 can instead be perfused by the LCX, if this artery is of the dominant type (observed in 10% of patients). At least part of segment 15 is perfused by the LAD if the LAD is long. Parts of segments 5, 11, and 16, via the posterolateral branches, are on certain occasions perfused by the RCA, if it is very dominant. Lastly, the RCA perfuses segment 17 if the LAD is very short. The AV node is usually perfused by the AV node artery, a branch of the posterior descending.

Circumflex coronary artery

The LCX artery perfuses most of the lateral wall – the anterior basal part (segment 6), and the mid and low parts shared with the LAD (segments 12 and 16) and often the entire inferior part of the lateral wall (segments 5 and 11) unless the RCA is very dominant. It also perfuses, especially if it is the dominant artery, a large part of the inferior wall, especially segment 4, on occasions, segment 10, and even part of segment 15 and the apex (segment 17).

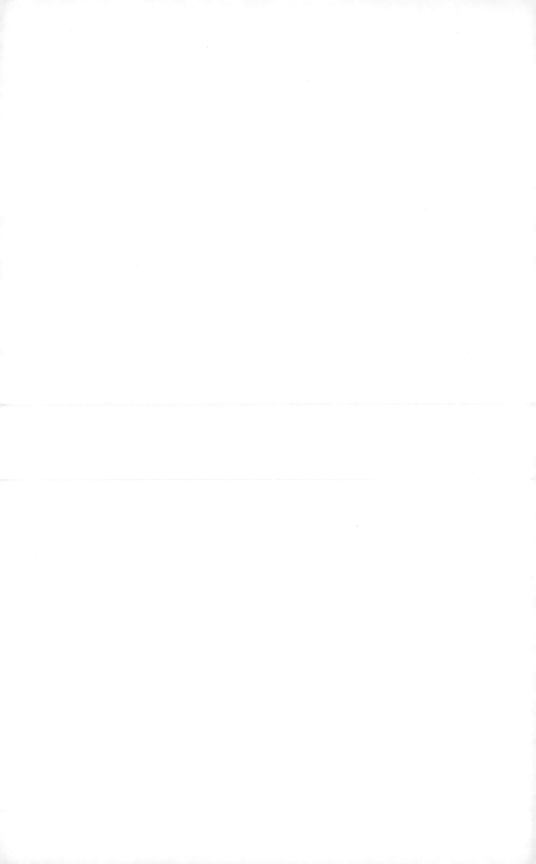

The ECG changes in ST elevation-myocardial infarction

STEMI-type myocardial infarction usually occurs in patients in whom the coronary occlusion is frequently complete or nearly complete and perfusion of the ventricular segments is severely compromised. After the complete occlusion, the ischemia occurs first in the subendocardium producing a taller T wave, but the ischemia soon becomes transmural and homogeneous (ST elevation). With persistent occlusion of an epicardial coronary artery the ST elevation evolves from an initial concave upward to a convex upward pattern. Finally, this is usually followed by a Q wave of necrosis and an inverted T wave (Figure 8).

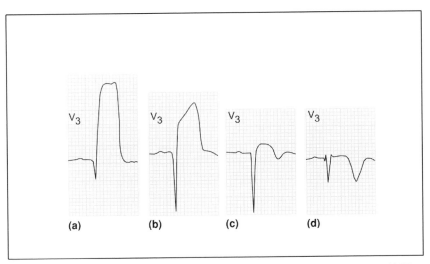

Figure 8 V₃ lead: Evolution of QRS and ST/T morphologies in STEMI due to occlusion of LAD. (a) Few minutes; (b) 1 hour; (c) 1 day; (d) 1 week.

CHAPTER 3

The concept of injury vector: direct and reciprocal changes

In the course of ST elevation-myocardial infarction (STEMI), ST-segment depression is frequently recorded in leads registering electrical signals from walls of the heart opposite to the area at risk (**reciprocal patterns**). These changes in the ST-segment are seen in leads other than those used for the diagnosis of STEMI. When the injury is transmural, the precordial leads indicate the left anterior descending coronary artery (LAD) is occluded and the inferior leads indicate the left circumflex coronary artery (LCX) or right coronary artery (RCA) are occluded. However, when the transmural injury occurs principally in the inferobasal segment of the inferior wall and/or in the lateral wall (basal and mid-posterior segments of the lateral wall), which occurs in some cases of LCX occlusion, the ST-segment elevation is seen in the posterior thoracic leads. ST-segment depression recorded in the V_{1-3} leads is a "mirror pattern" and is accompanied by ST elevation in inferior and/or V_{5-6} leads that may be smaller than the ST depression in V_{1-3}. Such patients with LCX occlusion are experiencing STEMI and should receive reperfusion therapy (see Case 1, p. 61). On the other hand, in a few cases of RCA proximal to the RV branches or when the RCA is very short, the ST elevation in V_{1-3} may be more striking than in the inferior leads.

All this, which is of great interest for identifying the culprit coronary artery is based on the fact that the injury vector is oriented towards the injured area and generates ST-segment elevation in the leads facing the vector's head and ST-segment depression in the leads facing the vector's tail (opposed leads) (Figures 9–11). Therefore, the **injury vector direction** is determined by the myocardial area at risk, which will be different according to the occluded artery and the site of the occlusion.

In Figures 9–11, it may be seen that ST-segment changes in reciprocal leads permits one to determine (a) whether the occlusion located in the LAD is proximal or distal to the first diagonal branch (Figure 9), (b) whether the occlusion is located in the RCA or in the LCX (Figure 10), and (c) whether the occlusion is proximal or distal to the first septal branch (S_1) (Figure 11).

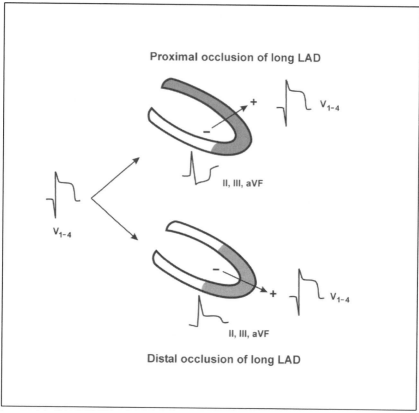

Figure 9 When evaluating a patient with STEMI with ST-segment elevation in precordial leads (V_{1-2} to V_{4-6}), we can strongly suggest that the occluded artery is the LAD. The correlation of the ST-segment elevation in V_{1-2} to V_{4-6} with the ST morphology in II, III, and aVF allows us to know if it is an occlusion proximal or distal to D_1. If it is proximal, the involved muscular mass in the anterior wall is large and the injury vector is directed forward and upward, even though there can be an evident inferior wall compromise if the LAD is long. This explains the negativity recorded in II, III, and aVF since these leads face the tail of the injury vector. On the contrary, when the involved myocardial mass in the anterior wall is smaller, because it is an occlusion distal to D_1, and the LAD is quite long, the injury vector in this U-shaped infarction (inferoanterior) is directed anteriorly, but somewhat downward, and so it generally produces slight ST-segment elevation in II, III, and aVF because these leads face the head of the injury vector (see Figures 17 and 19).

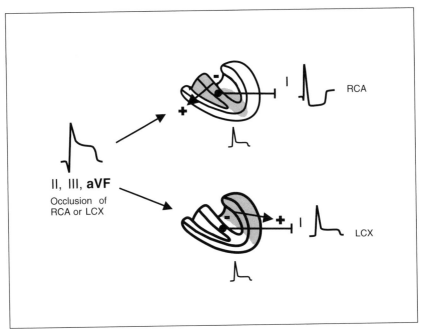

Figure 10 In a STEMI with ST-segment elevation present in II, III, and aVF, the study of the ST elevation and depression in different leads facilitates identification of the occluded artery (RCA or LCX) and even the site of the occlusion and its anatomical characteristics (dominance, etc). For example, in this figure we can see that if ST-segment depression exists in lead I, it means that this lead is facing the tail of the injury vector that is directed to the right, and therefore the occlusion is located in the RCA. On the contrary, when the occlusion is located in the LCX, lead I faces the injury vector head, and in this case it is directed somewhat to the left and will be recorded as ST-segment elevation in lead I. Therefore, checking the ST deviation in lead I may give a clue as to as to the location of the culprit artery (see Figure 37).

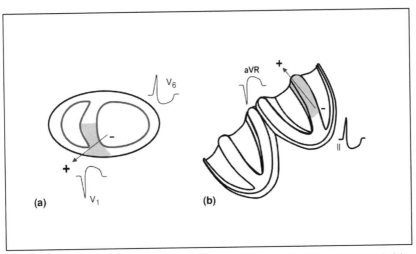

Figure 11 In the case of high septal involvement due to LAD occlusion before the take-off of the S_1 branch, the injured area generates an injury vector directed in the FP (b) and HP (a) upward, to the right, and forward. This explains ST elevation in aVR and V_1 and ST depression in the inferior leads, especially II and V_6 (see Figure 13).

CHAPTER 4

Clinical interpretation and significance of ST changes

In order to correctly stratify the risk in a patient having an ST elevation-myocardial infarction (STEMI), the characteristics of ST changes in the admission ECG could be used as follows: (a) to **check the elevation and depression in the different leads**, which allows one to localize the site of coronary occlusion and the area at risk; (b) to **sum up in millimeters the ST-segment deviations**, which helps to quantify, with limitations (see later), the area at risk; and (c) to **assess the morphology of the ST-segment elevation**, which gives additional information related to prognosis. We will focus our attention on the importance of checking the ST deviations in order to assess the location of the occlusion (Bayés de Luna & Fiol 2006, Birnbaum et al. 1994, 1996, Gorgels et al. 2003, Martinez-Dolz et al. 2002, Prieto et al. 2002, Sclarowsky 1999). Despite the advantages that this approach represents, we would like to emphasize certain limitations, especially in relation to the transient nature of some of the ST deviations and the small number of patients studied in some series.

Location of the occlusion and risk stratification: the role of deviations of the ST-segment

In the classical ECG assessment of a STEMI, the leads with electrocardiographic ST elevation are used to diagnose the location of the injury, but not much information is sought regarding where the occlusion is located and the size of the area at risk.

We will comment in the following pages how we may obtain all this information through the adequate and careful study of the correlations between coronary angiography and the deviations of the ST-segment that are registered according to the projection of the injury vector in the positive and negative hemifields of different leads. All this information will permit us to determine the location of the area at risk due to the occluded artery and may help in deciding on the need for and even the urgency of performing a primary percutaneous coronary intervention (PCI) (Bayés de Luna & Fiol 2006, Gorgels et al. 2003, Gallik et al.1995, Sclarowsky 1999).

Now we will discuss two different aspects of these correlations: (1) **how to identify the area at risk and the corresponding ECG based on the location of the occluded artery**, and (2) **performing the opposite exercise, that is, how one can identify the area at risk and the occlusion site based on the ECG findings**. The clinicians receiving a patient with chest pain in the Emergency

Department should carry out this second exercise promptly because the ECG changes appear much earlier than biomarker elevation.

1. From the occluded artery to the area at risk and the corresponding electrocardiographic abnormality

Table 1 shows the most frequent patterns of STEMI; the site of occlusion in the coronary circulation, the involved myocardial segments, and the spatial location of the injury vector are shown in this section. **The correlation of the injury vector with the positive and negative hemifields of the different leads explains the ST-segment elevations or depressions that are seen in different situations** (Fiol et al. 2004b; Wellens et al. 2003).

The left ventricle is divided into two zones: anteroseptal and inferolateral (Figure 7a). The involvement of the anteroseptal zone corresponds to cases with occlusion of the left anterior descending coronary artery (LAD) and its branches (Table 1), while the involvement of the inferolateral zone corresponds to the occlusion of the right coronary artery (RCA) and the left circumflex coronary artery (LCX) (Table 1). We will study 12 different locations of coronary occlusions that define 12 areas at risk, 6 in the anteroseptal zone (Table 1a) and 6 in the inferolateral zone (Table 1b). The ECG patterns that match these different areas will be discussed.

Anteroseptal zone: occlusion of the LAD and its branches

The LAD occlusion (Table 1, from 1 to 6) may be located (a) above the first diagonal (D_1) and the first septal (S_1) branches; (b) above the D_1, branch but distal to the S_1 branch; (c) below both the S_1 and D_1 branches; (d) above the S_1 branch but distal to the D_1 branch; (e) LAD occlusion including the diagonal branches but not the septal branches or just a selective D_1–D_2 occlusion; and (f) LAD occlusion involving the septal branches but not the diagonal branches or rarely a selective S_1–S_2 occlusion (Bayés de Luna & Fiol 2006, Bayés de Luna & Malik 2005, Birnbaum et al. 1994, Engelen et al. 1999, Sclarowsky 1999).

Occlusion above the D_1 and S_1 branches[1]

When the occlusion is located above the D_1 and S_1 branches (Figure 12a), the **area at risk** is large and without treatment could lead to an extensive anterior infarction. **The area affected by the occlusion** may be seen in Figure 12b, and its projection onto a polar map is shown in Figure 12c. The most affected segments are 1, 2, 7, 8, 13, 14, and 17, and part of segments 12, 16, 3, 9, and 15.

In this case, the **injury vector** is directed anteriorly and upward, and somewhat to the right or the left, depending on whether septal – the most frequent – or lateral involvement predominates (Figure 12d). The projection of this vector in the positive and negative hemifields of different leads explains the ST-segment elevation from V_1 to V_4, and in aVR. When the involvement

---

[1] Sometimes these are the second septal or diagonal branches because the anatomically S_1 or D_1 are very short and narrow.

Table 1 STEMI: correlations between the ECG abnormalities, the injured myocardial area, and the place of coronary occlusion.

a Most prominent pattern of **ST elevation in precordial leads I and aVL*** (anteroseptal zone)			b Most prominent pattern of **ST elevation in inferior and/or lateral leads**† (inferolateral zone)		
Occluded artery	Injured myocardial area (see Figure 7)	Leads with ST changes	Occluded artery (RCA vs LCX)	Injured myocardial wall (see Figure 7)	Leads with ST changes
1. LAD occlusion proximal to D_1 and S_1	Extensive anteroseptal zone (especially 1, 2, 7, 8, 13, 14, 16, and 17 segments)	• ST↑ in V_1 to V_{4-5} and aVR • ST↓ in II, III, aAVF, and often V_{5-6}	7. RCA occlusion proximal to the RV branches	Same as type 8 plus injury of RV	• ST↑ in II, III, and aVF with III > II • ST↓ in I, aVL • ST↑ in V_4R with T+ • ST isoelectric or elevated in V_1
2. LAD occlusion proximal to D_1 but distal to S_1	Anteroseptal or extensive anterior (especially 1, 7, 13, 14, 16, and 17 segments)	• ST↑ in V_2 to V_{5-6}, I, VL • ST↓ in II, III, and aVF	8. RCA occlusion distal to the RV branches	Inferior wall and/or the inferior part of the septum (especially 3, 4, 9, 10, 14, and 15 segments)	• ST↑ in II, III, and aVF with III > II • ST↓ in I and aVL • ST↓ in V_{1-3} but if affected zone is very small, almost no ST↓ in V_{1-2}
3. LAD occlusion distal to D_1 and S_1	Apical (especially 13, 14, 15, 16, 17, and part of 7 and 8 segments)	• ST↑ in V_2 to V_{4-5} • ST↑ or = in II, III, and aVF If LAD is short less evident changes	9. Very dominant RCA occlusion	Great part of inferolateral zone (especially 3, 4, 5, 9, 10, 11, 14, 15, 16, and 17 segments). Injury of RV if RCA is proximally occluded	• ST↑ in II, III, aVF with III > II • ST↓ in V_{1-3} < ST ↑ in II, III, aVF. If the RCA is proximally occluded ST in V_{1-3} is = or ↑ • ST↓ in I and aVL with VL > V1 • ST ↑ in V_{5-6} ≥ 2 mm

(Continued)

Table 1 (*Continued*)

a Most prominent pattern of **ST elevation in precordial leads I and aVL** * (anteroseptal zone)

Occluded artery	Injured myocardial area (see Figure 7)	Leads with ST changes
4. LAD occlusion proximal to S_1 but distal to D_1	Anteroseptal (especially 2, 8, 13, 14, 15, 16, and 17 segments)	• ST↑ in V_1 to V_4, V_5, and aVR • ST↑ or = in II, III, and aVR • ST↓ in V_6
5. LAD suboclusion including D_1, but not S_1, or selective D_1 occlusion	Anterolateral limited (especially 7, 13, 12, and part of 1 and 16 segments)	• ST↑ in I, aVL, and sometimes V_2–V_{5-6} • ST↓ in II, III, aVF (III > II)
6. LAD suboclusion including S_1 but not D_1, or selective S_1 occlusion	Septal (especially 2, 8, and sometimes part of 1, 3, 9, 14 segments)	• ST↑ in V_{1-2}, aVR • ST↓ in I, II, III, aVF, V_6 (II > III)

b Most prominent pattern of **ST elevation in inferior and/or lateral leads** † (inferolateral zone)

Occluded artery (RCA vs LCX)	Injured myocardial wall (see Figure 7)	Leads with ST changes
10. LCX occlusion proximal to first OM branches	Lateral wall and inferior wall, especially the inferobasal segment (espe- cially 4, 5, 6, 10, 11, 12 segments)	• ST↓ in V_{1-3} (mirror image) greater than ST↑ in inferior leads • ST↑ in II, III, aVF (II > III) • Usually, ST↑ in V_{5-6} • ST↑ in I, VL (I > VL)
11. First OM occlusion	Lateral wall (especially 6, 12, and 16 segments)	• Often ST↑ in I, aVL, V_{5-6} and/or in II, III, aVF. Usually slight • Often slight ST↓ in V_{1-3}
12. Very dominant LCX occlusion	Great part of inferolateral zone (especially 3, 4, 5, 6, 9, 10, 11, 12, 15 and 16 segments)	• ST↑ in II, III, aVF (II ≥ III) often greater than ST↓ in V_{1-3} • The ST may be depressed in aVL but usually not in I • ST elevation in V_{5-6} is sometimes very evident

* See Figure 36.
† See Figure 37.

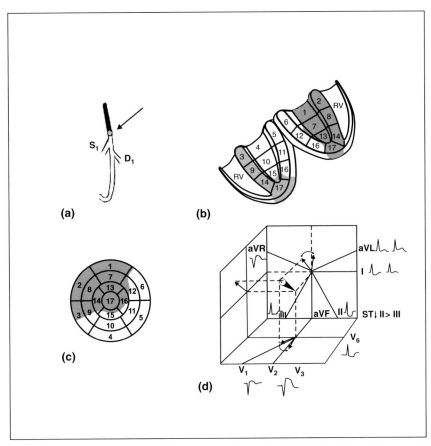

Figure 12 STEMI due to LAD occlusion proximal to D_1 and S_1: (a) site of occlusion; (b) myocardial area at risk in gray; (c) affected segments are marked in gray in "bull's-eye" projection; (d) injury vector in an acute phase and its projection in frontal, horizontal, and sagittal planes. The injury vector is usually directed somewhat to the right (see arrows in FP and HP projection) because the occlusion is proximal not only to D_1 but also to S_1. This explains, by the correlation of the projection of the injury vector in FP and HP, the deviations of the ST segment in different leads (see text).

of the anterolateral area is predominant, the ST elevation is also seen in aVL and often in I because the injury vector falls in the positive hemifield of aVL and on the border of positive hemifield of I (around $-90°$). The larger the ST-segment elevation in aVL (anterolateral involvement), the lesser the changes in aVR (anteroseptal involvement) and vice versa. ST-segment depression occurs in the inferior leads especially in II and also in V_{5-6} because the anteroseptal compromise is usually predominant over the anterolateral compromise and the injury vector is directed somewhat to the right and upward (Figures 12d and 13). In our experience (Bayés de Luna & Fiol 2006), ST-segment depression in the inferior wall (III + aVF $\geq$ 2.5 mm) is quite suggestive of a proximal occlusion of LAD above D_1 (Figure 9), while ST-segment depression in V_6

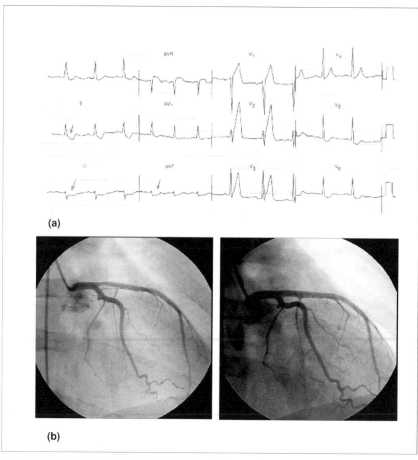

(a)

(b)

Figure 13 (a) The ECG of STEMI due to LAD occlusion proximal to D_1 and S_1 in the hyperacute phase. ST elevation from V_1 to V_3 and also in aVR is recorded. Also, ST depression in II, III, aVF (more in II) and in V_{5-6} is evident. This may be explained by the LAD occlusion proximal not only to D_1 but also to S_1, which as a consequence provokes an injury vector directed forward, upward, and somewhat to the right, and therefore falls in the negative hemifield of V_6 and sometimes V_5 and I, and in the positive hemifield of aVR and V_1. (b) Coronary angiography before (left) and after (right) reperfusion.

with ST-segment elevation in aVR and V_1 is quite specific for occlusion above the S_1 branch (ST↑ VR and V_1 + ST↓ V_6 > 0) (Figures 11 and 36).

Minimal ST-segment elevation in V_1 in some cases of high septal involvement (occlusion above S_1) may be explained by the fact that the superior septal portion is perfused not only by the LAD, but also by the RCA (double perfusion).

A typical electrocardiographic example of this type of STEMI is shown in Figure 13a, along with its correlation with the coronary angiogram (Figure 13b) before and after fibrinolytic therapy.

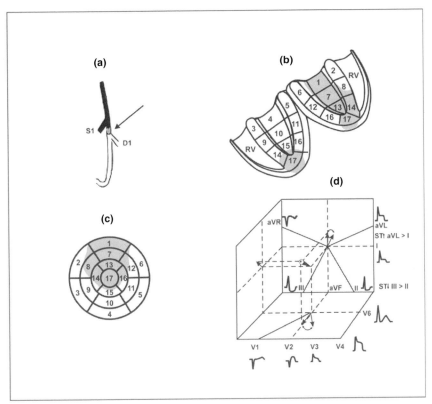

Figure 14 STEMI due to LAD occlusion proximal to D_1 but distal to S_1: (a) site of occlusion; (b) myocardial area at risk; (c) "bull's-eye" polar map with affected segments. The involvement of the apex will depend on the presence of a short or long LAD. Nevertheless, one should remember that the apex is generally affected as the LAD is long in approximately 80% of cases; (d) injury vector in the acute phase is directed forward, upward, and somewhat to the left (see arrows in the FP and HP projection), as the high part of septum is not affected. The correlation projection of the injury vector in different hemifields explains the ST changes (see text).

Occlusion proximal to D_1 branch but distal to the S_1 branch
When the occlusion is above D_1 but not S_1 (Figure 14a), the **area at risk** could lead to an anterior infarction, with extension to the mid-low part of the septal and lateral anterior walls (due to the proximal occlusion of the D_1 branch). Remember that the upper anterior part of the lateral wall is perfused by the LCX. When the S_1 branch is small, the area of the septal wall involved will be larger. Without the initiation of urgent reperfusion therapy, necrosis of the septal wall could be large (all the septal branches distal to S_1) and consequently could lead to an extensive infarction (Figure 14b). The area involved by the occlusion and its projection onto a polar map is shown in Figure 14c. The more affected segments are 1, 7, 13, 14, and 17, but also part of segment 12, and sometimes part of segments 2, 8, 15, and 16.

In this case, the **injury vector** is directed anteriorly, upward, and somewhat to the left (Figure 14d). The projection of the injury vector in different positive and negative hemifields of different leads of the frontal plane (FP) and the horizontal plane (HP) explains the ST-segment elevation from V_{2-3} to V_{5-6} but not usually in V_1, because the projection of this vector in the HP falls frequently a little to the left, in the limit of the negative hemifield of V_1. Also these correlations explain the ST elevation in lead I and especially in aVL, and the ST-segment depression in the inferior leads (III + aVF $\geq$ 2.5 mm) (Figures 14 and 15). Usually, more ST-segment depression is seen in III than in II, since lead III is opposed to aVL, and therefore the injury vector falls more in the negative hemifield of III and this lead faces the injury vector tail more directly.

A typical example of this type of STEMI is shown in Figure 15a, along with its correlation with the coronary angiogram (Figure 15b) before and after fibrinolytic therapy.

Occlusion distal to the S_1 and D_1 branches
When the occlusion is located distal to S_1 and D_1 (Figure 16a), the **area at risk** involves the inferior third of the left ventricle, with almost invariably some inferior involvement and only low-lateral involvement (apical infarction). In Figure 16b the area affected can be observed, and in Figure 16c a polar map of that area is shown. The more affected segments are 13, 14, 15, 16, and 17, and sometimes part of segments 7, 8, 12, and 16.

In this case, the **injury vector** is directed anteriorly and often rather to the left (to the apex), but not upward. When the LAD is long, it may perfuse a large portion of the inferior wall and then the injury vector is also directed downward (Figure 16d). The projection of this vector in the FP and HP explains the ST-segment elevation from V_{2-3} to V_{4-6} but not in V_1 and/or aVR, because usually the injury vector falls in the limit of positive and negative hemifields of V_1 and clearly in the negative hemifield of aVR. Due to downward direction of this vector there is usually slight ST-segment depression in aVR and elevation in II, III, and VF (II > III), because usually the injury vector is directed downward and a little to the left. When the LAD is short, the infarction distal to S_1 and D_1 is small, and no changes are typically seen in the FP, or if they occur, they consist of just a slight ST-segment elevation or depression.

A typical electrocardiographic example of this STEMI is shown in Figure 17a, along with its coronary angiographic correlation before and after fibrinolytic therapy (Figure 17b).

Also, the ST-segment elevation is seen in the precordial and inferior leads in the presence of a STEMI due to the very proximal occlusion of the RCA. In this case the ST-segment elevation usually is $V_1 > V_{3-4}$, while in a STEMI due to the distal occlusion of the LAD the opposite occurs (i.e., the ST-segment elevation is $V_1 < V_{3-4}$). Table 2 shows the ECG criteria that allow the culprit artery (proximal RCA or distal LAD) to be differentiated in the case of ST elevation in the precordial and inferior leads (see p. 50).

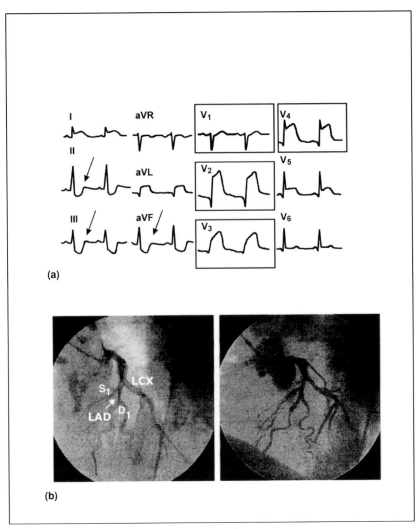

Figure 15 (a) The ECG of STEMI due to occlusion of the LAD proximal to D_1 but distal to S_1. Observe the ST elevation from V_2 to V_5 with ST depression in II, III, and VF. Nevertheless, there is neither ST elevation in V_1 and aVR nor ST depression in V_6, because the occlusion is distal to S_1, and the injury vector may fall in the limit between the positive and negative hemifields of aVR and V_1 and in the positive hemifield of V_{5-6}. (b) Coronary angiography before (left) and after (right) reperfusion. The arrow indicates the place of occlusion.

Occlusion proximal to the S_1 branch but distal to the D_1 branch
When the occlusion is located above the S_1 but not the D_1 (Figure 18), which rarely occurs (<5% of the STEMI), the **area at risk** could lead to an anteroseptal infarction. The area at risk is more extensive when the D_1 branch is quite small and the D_2 branch is large. However, usually more septal and anterior than

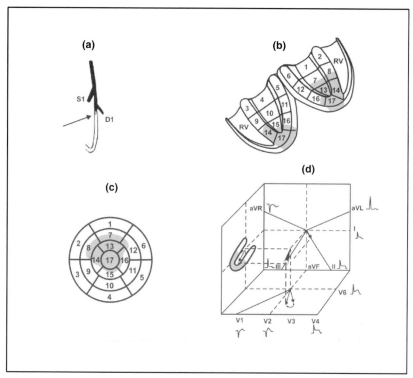

Figure 16 STEMI due to occlusion of a long LAD distal to D_1 and S_1: (a) site of occlusion; (b) myocardial area at risk; (c) affected segments in "bull's-eye" projection; (d) injury vector is directed forward and a little to the left, and somehow downward, resulting in ST-segment elevations in FP and HP leads, but clearly with more important projection (ST elevation) in the HP precordial leads than in the FP (inferior leads) (see text).

lateral involvement is seen (Figure 18b and c). The area more usually involved by the occlusion may be seen in Figure 18b, and its projection onto a polar map is shown in Figure 18c. The more affected segments are 2, 8, 13, 14, 16, and 17, and generally part of segments 3, 7, 9, and 15. Usually, segment 1 and part of segment 7 are spared because they are protected by the occlusion of the LAD distal to D_1.

The **injury vector** is directed anteriorly, to the right and sometimes downward, especially if the LAD is long and wraps around the apex, affecting part of the inferior wall; then, if the anterior wall is not greatly affected because the occlusion occurs below a large D_1, the involvement of the inferior wall can turn out to be more important than the involvement of the anterior wall. The projection of this injury vector in the positive and negative hemifields of different leads of the FP and HP explains the ST-segment elevation from V_1 to V_4 and that the isoelectric or elevated ST-segment in the inferior leads is more evident

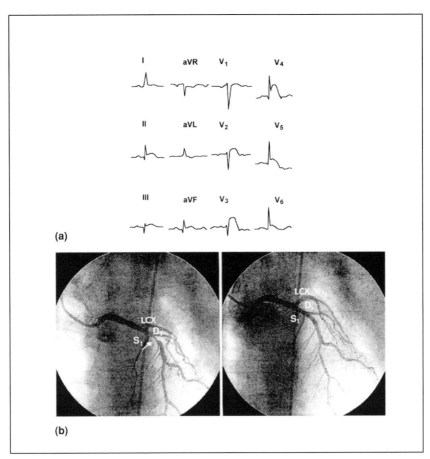

(a)

(b)

Figure 17 (a) The ECG of STEMI in the case of LAD occlusion distal to D_1 and S_1. Observe the ST elevation from V_2 to V_{5-6} with ST somehow elevated in II, III, and aVF. The elevation of ST in the HP leads is greater because the projection of the injury vector on the HP is much larger than on the FP (see Figure 16). (b) Coronary angiography before (left) and after (right) reperfusion. The arrow indicates the place of occlusion.

Table 2 ST elevation in precordial leads (especially V_1 to V_{3-4}) and inferior leads (II, III, VF).

Leads	RCA (proximal RCA)	LAD[†]
V_1 to V_{3-4}	Usually ST↑ ($V_1 > V_{3-4}$)*	Usually ST↑ ($V_{3-4} > V_1$)
Inferior leads	Usually ST↑ greater than that in precordial leads	ST↑ usually much lesser than that in precordial leads
I and aVL	ST depresssion (usually the sum $\geq$ 5 mm)	Usually not ST depression especially in I

* In exceptional cases of very dominant RCA occluded proximally, the ST elevation may be seen in all the precordial leads. In V_1 to V_{3-4} due to proximal occlusion and in V_{5-6} due to very dominant RCA (local injury vector) (see Figure 28 and Case 12).
[†] Distal occlusion of long LAD or distal occlusion of LAD + total occlusion of RCA with colateral vessels.

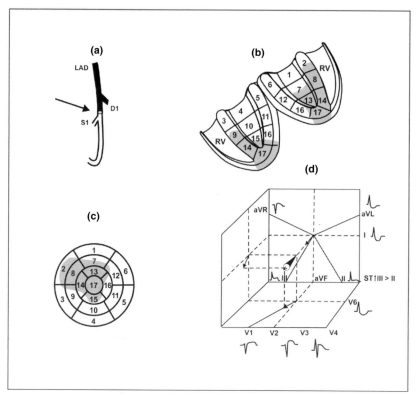

Figure 18 STEMI due to LAD occlusion proximal to S_1 but distal to D_1: (a) site of occlusion; (b) myocardial area at risk; (c) "bull's-eye" polar map with affected segments; (d) injury vector directed to the right and forward due to occlusion proximal to S_1. In the case of a long LAD also affecting the inferior wall, the vector can be directed downward. This is due to the relatively small myocardial area of the anterior wall affected in the case of occlusion distal to D_1. This explains the ST elevation from V_1 to V_{3-4} and in general also the ST elevation in II, III, and VF (due to occlusion distal to D_1). Occlusion proximal to S_1 explains the ST elevation in aVR and V_1 and the ST depression in V_6, I, and aVL because the injury vector is directed to the right in this case and falls in the positive hemifield of aVR and V_1 and in the negative hemifield of I, aVL, and V_6 (see text).

in III than in II because the injury vector is directed a little downward and to the right (III > II). An ST-segment depression is seen in V_6 and aVL, and sometimes an ST-segment elevation in aVR (Figure 18d).

A typical electrocardiographic example of this type of STEMI is shown in Figure 19.

LAD occlusion involving the diagonal branches but not the septal branches, or selective occlusion of the D_1 branch
In this case (Figure 20a) the **area at risk** usually involves the mid-low anterior wall and part of the mid- and often low-lateral wall, but not the basal portion of the lateral wall that is perfused by the LCX. In Figure 20b and c the involved

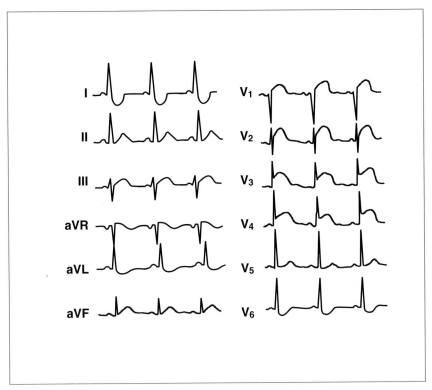

Figure 19 A typical example of a STEMI with LAD occlusion proximal to S_1 and distal to D_1. Observe the ST elevation in II, III, and VF due to occlusion being distal to D_1, and ST elevation in aVR and in V_1 to V_4, with depression in V_6 since the occlusion is proximal to S_1.

myocardial area and the polar map of that area are shown. The more affected segments are 7 and 13, and generally part of segments 1, 12, and 16 (Birnbaum et al. 1996).

The **injury vector** is directed upward, to the left and forward (Figure 20d), which, according to the correlations of the injury vector and projection in positive and negative hemifields of different leads, explains the ST-segment elevation in I, aVL, and, sometimes, in the precordial leads, especially from V_{2-3} to V_{5-6}, and the ST-segment depression in II, III, and VF (III > II). The presence of slight ST depression in V_{2-3} may be seen in some cases of multiple-vessel occlusion (D_1 + LCX or RCA). Classically it was considered that the aVL lead faces the high-lateral wall. However, the presence of ST elevation in acute phase in aVL or QS in chronic phase without Q in V_{5-6}, as is seen in this case, is explained by the involvement of the middle part of the anterior and lateral walls perfused by D_1 and not by the involvement of the high-lateral wall that is perfused by LCX (Bayés de Luna & Fiol 2006).

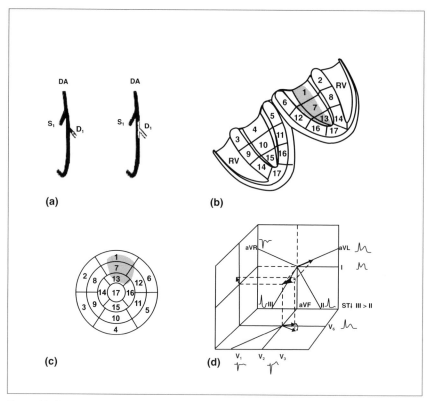

Figure 20 STEMI due to selective occlusion of D_1 or occlusion of the LAD involving the diagonal but not the septal branches: (a) site of occlusion; (b) myocardial area at risk; (c) "bull's-eye" polar map with affected segments; (d) injury vector with its projection in frontal, horizontal, and sagittal planes as well as corresponding ECG morphologies. The projection of the vector in the FP around $-30°$ explains the ST elevation in I and VL and the ST depression in inferior leads, especiallly III (see text).

An electrocardiographic example of this type of STEMI with QS in aVL in the chronic phase is shown in Figure 21.

LAD occlusion involving the septal branches but not the diagonal branches or, more rarely, selective occlusion of the S_1 branch

In this case the **area at risk** involves more or less extensively, according to the number of septal branches involved, the septal wall with occasionally certain extension toward the anterior wall. The occlusion rarely is located in the S_1 or S_2 branches (Figure 22a). In Figure 22b and c the involved area and the polar map are shown. The most affected segments are 2, 8, and sometimes part of segments 1, 3, 9, and 14.

The **injury vector** is directed anteriorly, upward, and to the right (Figure 22d), and therefore its projection in the positive and negative hemifields of different

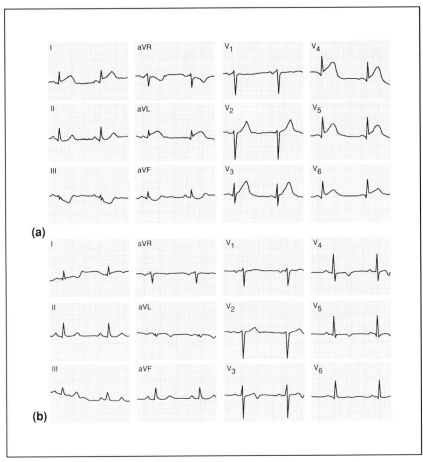

Figure 21 (a) The typical ECG pattern of STEMI due to D_1 occlusion. Observe the ST elevation in I, aVL, V_3 to V_6 and ST depression in II, III, aVF. (b) The same case is shown in the chronic phase with QS in aVL and low-voltage R in lead I.

leads of the FP and HP explains the ST-segment elevation in V_1, V_2, and aVR, with ST depression in II, III, aVF (II > III), and V_6 and lack of ST elevation in aVL.

In Figure 23 an example of a STEMI secondary to occlusion of a large S_1 branch during a PCI procedure is shown (Tamura et al. 1991).

Inferolateral zone: RCA or LCX occlusion

When the RCA occlusion is quite proximal and compromises the right marginal branches that perfuse the right ventricle (RV), the infarction also affects most of that ventricle. Along its final course it divides into two branches, the posteroseptal (directed toward the posterior septal wall) and the posterolateral (directed toward the inferior wall and, when it is quite dominant, to the

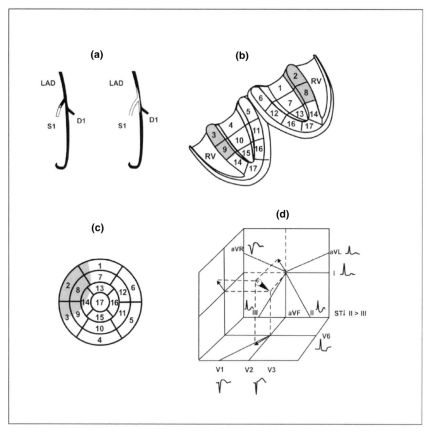

Figure 22 STEMI due to subocclusion of the LAD affecting the septal branches but not the diagonal branches. In exceptional cases only selective S_1 or S_2 occlusion may be found: (a) site of the occlusion; (b) myocardial area at risk; (c) affected segments in a bull's-eye projection; (d) injury vector projected on frontal, horizontal, and sagittal planes with corresponding ECG morphologies. Observe how this vector directed upward, forward, and rightward explains the ST elevation in V_{1-4} and aVR and ST depression in inferior leads, I and V_6, and lack of ST elevation in aVL (see text).

posterior part of the lateral wall) (Figures 1 and 7). We will comment on the ECG abnormalities when the occlusion is located proximal and distal to the RV branches and also in the case of a very dominant RCA (Table 1b, from 7 to 12).

The LCX traveling along the high-lateral aspect of the left ventricle curves backward and gives rise to one or more obtuse marginal (OM) branches perfusing the greatest part of the lateral wall and especially the basal part of the inferior wall (Figures 1 and 7). When it is quite dominant, it also perfuses the inferior portion of that wall and even a portion of the inferior part of the septal wall. We will comment on the ECG abnormalities when the occlusion is located before the take-off of the OM, in the OM, and in the case of a very dominant LCX.

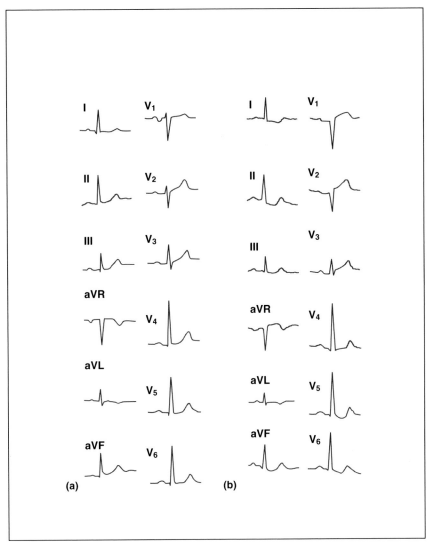

Figure 23 (a) Control ECG. (b) A typical ECG pattern in occlusion of a large S_1 artery during a PCI procedure with the involvement of the basal and probably also the mid-septal part (adapted from Tamura et al. 1991). Observe the ST depression in II and V_6 and ST elevation in aVR and V_1.

RCA occlusion proximal to the RV branches
When the RCA occlusion is proximal to the bulk of the arterial supply to the RV (Figure 24a), the **area at risk** involves not only the inferior wall and a portion of the inferior part of the septal wall, but also the RV. In Figure 24b and c the involved myocardial area and the polar map in the case of a short RCA or balanced dominance are shown. The more affected segments are 3, 4, 9, and 10, and part of segments 14 and 15.

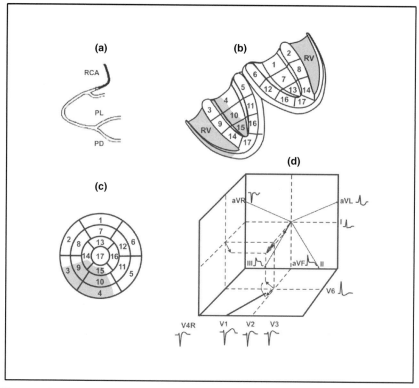

Figure 24 STEMI due to RCA occlusion proximal to the right ventricular marginal branch in the case of balanced dominance: (a) site of occlusion; (b) myocardial area at risk; (c) polar map in "bull's-eye" projection with the most affected segments marked in gray; (d) injury vector projected on frontal, horizontal, and sagittal planes with corresponding ECG morphologies. Observe how the injury vector due to RV involvement is directed downward but more forward than in the case of RCA occlusion distal to the RV branches. This vector falls in the limit of positive hemifield of V_1 or inside (between $+100°$ and $+200°$) and this explains that ST in V_1 and even V_{2-3} may be isoelectric or even positive (see text).

Due to the right ventricular extension, the **injury vector** that is always directed downward, posteriorly, and to the right in the cases of infarction secondary to occlusion of the RCA is directed less posteriorly and more to the right than the direction it would have taken if the RV were not involved (compare Figures 24d and 26d). The projection of the injury vector in the positive and negative hemifields of different leads of the FP and HP explains the ST-segment elevation in II, III, and VF (III > II), and the ST-segment depression in V_6, I, and aVL (aVL > I). It also explains why the ST-segment depression in V_{1-3} is generally absent in the case of occlusion proximal to the RV marginal branches, or why even ST-segment elevation may be recorded, especially in V_1 (Fiol et al. 2004a). For the same reason, ST-segment elevation may be recorded in V_3R and V_4R. Lead V_4R is useful during the hyperacute phase to distinguish

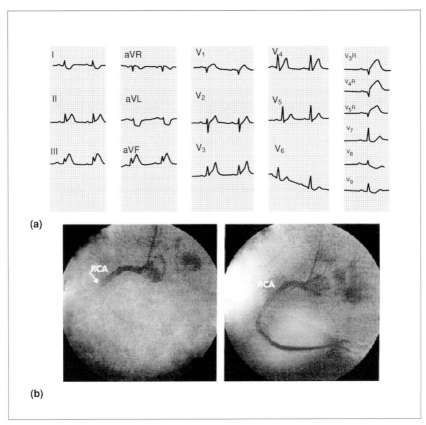

(a)

(b)

Figure 25 (a) The ECG in the case of STEMI due to proximal RCA occlusion with RV involvement. Observe ST elevation in II, III, VF (with III > II), because the projection of the vector in the FP falls more in the positive hemifield of III than of II. The same vector explains the ST depression in I and isoelectric or elevated ST in V_{1-3} as well as ST elevation with positive T wave in V_3R–V_4R leads. (b) Coronary angiography before (left) and after (right) reperfusion. The arrow indicates the place of occlusion.

an occlusion of the RCA proximal to the RV branch from an occlusion of the RCA distal to the RV branch and from an occlusion of the LCX (Figure 37) (Wellens et al. 2003). However, ST-segment changes in these leads are quite transient and often are not recorded. Therefore, V_1 (isoelectric or elevated ST-segment) has been shown to be equally useful (Fiol et al. 2004a) for detecting an occlusion proximal to the RV branch. It also has the advantage of not requiring the recording of additional leads. Figure 25 shows a similar morphology of ST elevation in V_1 and $V_{3-4}R$.

In the case of RCA occlusion proximal to the RV branches, sometimes if the RCA is very short with involvement exclusively of the RV (Finn 2003), ST-segment elevation may be seen from V_1 to V_{3-4}, but the elevation in V_1 is greater than in V_{3-4} ($V_1 > V_{3-4}$), the opposite to that which occurs in LAD occlusion distal to the S_1 and D_1 branches. In these latter cases, ST-segment elevation may also be seen in the precordial and inferior leads, but with ST elevation in V_{3-4} greater than that that in V_1 (Sadananden et al. 2003). The ECG criteria that support occlusion of the RCA or the LAD in the case of ST elevation in both groups of leads, inferior and precordial, are shown in Table 2.

A typical electrocardiographic example of this type of STEMI is shown in Figure 25a, along with its correlation with the coronary angiogram (Figure 25b) before and after a primary percutaneous transluminal coronary anigoplasty.

The lack of apparent ST depression in V_{1-3} may also be observed in the occurrence of a small inferior MI due to a very distal occlusion of a nondominant RCA. In these cases, because the area at risk is very small, the ST-segment elevation is not very apparent in II, III, and VF.

RCA occlusion distal to main arterial supply to the RV branches
When the occlusion is located in the RCA distal to the RV branches (Figure 26a), in the case of balanced dominance the **area at risk** involves, if the occlusion is just after the RV branches, a part of the inferolateral zone similar to the case of occlusion proximal to the RV branches (see earlier). In Figure 26b and c the involved myocardial area and the polar map of that area are shown. The involved segments are 3, 4, 9, and 10 and part of segments 14 and 15. These cases never evolve toward a right ventricular infarction, since the main artery perfusing the RV branch is proximal to the occlusion.

The **injury vector** is directed downward, to the right (though less so than when the occlusion is proximal to the RV branches), and posteriorly, even though usually it is directed more downward than posteriorly. Although the segmentary left ventricular involvement may be greater than the involvement seen when the occlusion is located proximal to the RV branches, the direction of the injury vector is different in both cases, due to the RV involvement (compare Figures 24d and 26d). The projection of this vector in the positive and negative hemifields of different leads of the FP and HP explains why there is usually more ST-segment elevation in II, III, and VF (III > II) than ST-segment depression in V_{1-3} (projection vector in FP larger than in HP) (Figure 26d). Because the injury vector is directed to the right and downward, it is common that ST-segment depression is recorded in lead V_6, I, and even more in aVL because the injury vector falls within the negative hemifield of these leads but more in the negative hemifield of aVL.

A typical electrocardiographic example of this type of STEMI is shown in Figure 27.

Occlusion of a very dominant RCA
When the RCA is very dominant (Figure 28a), the **area at risk** involves a great part of the inferolateral zone, which includes a great part of the posterior septum, the inferior wall, and even the apex if the LAD is short, and a portion of the posterior and lower part of the lateral wall. The involved segments are 3, 4, 5, 9, 10, 11, 14, 15, and 16 (Figure 28b and c).

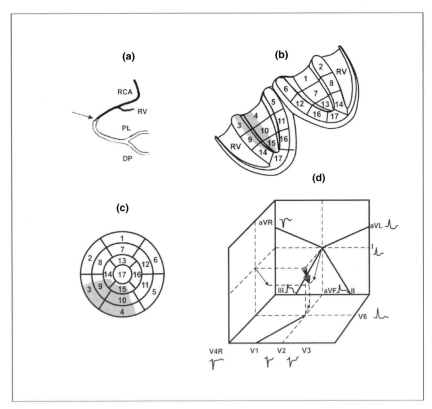

Figure 26 STEMI due to RCA occlusion after the RV branches (arrow). At the same degree of dominance (RCA vs LCX), the area at risk of the left ventricle may be the same as in the case of occlusion proximal to the RV branches. (a) Site of occlusion; (b) myocardial area at risk; (c) polar map in "bull's-eye" projection with the most affected segments marked in gray; (d) injury vector projected in frontal, horizontal, and sagittal planes is directed backward and somehow to the right but much less than in the case of RCA involving the RV branches. The injury vector in this case falls completely in the negative hemifield of V_{1-2}, and therefore the ST-segment will be depressed in these leads. As the RCA is not dominant, the ST-segment in V_6 is normal or slightly negative. Leads V_3R and V_4R show a positive T wave without ST elevation, as it occurs in cases of RCA occlusion distal to the RV branches.

The **injury vector** is directed downward and posteriorly and to the right. In the presence of occlusion proximal to the RV branches, the injury vector will be more directed to the right and even may fall in the positive hemifield of V_1 (see Figure 28d). This explains the ST being isoelectric or even having slight elevation in V_1 and sometimes also elevated in V_{2-4} (Figure 28d). However, the ST elevation in V_{5-6} (low inferolateral involvement) is explained by the presence of a local injury vector (Figure 28d). This local injury vector may be visible in V_{5-6} because of its proximity to the precordial leads. The influence of this local injury vector is more evident when the occlusion is below the RV branches. In the latter case, the injury vector is directed less rightward and does

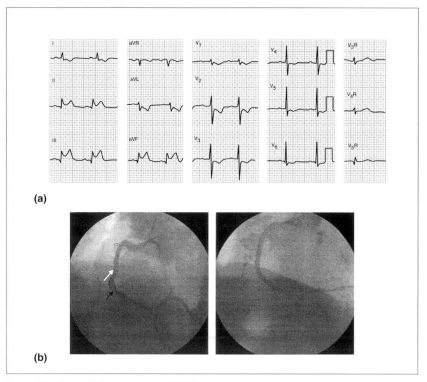

Figure 27 (a) The ECG in the case of STEMI due to RCA occlusion distal to the RV branches. Observe ST elevation in II, III, VF (III > II) with ST depression in I. There exists ST depression in right precordial leads (V_{1-2}). (b) Coronary angiography before (left) and after (right) reperfusion. The arrow indicates the place of occlusion.

not counterbalance the local injury vector as much. Therefore, the ST elevation in V_{5-6} is usually more visible in the absence of RV involvement.

In general in these cases the presence of ST elevation in II, III, and VF is very important, and if the occlusion is distal to the RV branches, the ST depression in V_{1-3} is also evident, although usually the ratio $\Sigma \uparrow ST$ in II, III, VF/$\Sigma \downarrow ST$ in V_{1-3} is greater than 1. The ST may be isoelectric or even positive in V_1 to V_{3-4} if the occlusion is above the RV branches, and as the ST may also be elevated in V_{5-6}; in exceptional cases of very dominant proximal RCA occlusion ST elevation in II, III, VF, and all precordial leads may be seen (see Case 12, Chapter 6). These cases have to be differentiated from LAD occlusion (see Table 2).

When the RCA is very dominant, ST-segment elevation ≥ 2 mm is usually seen in V_{5-6} (apical inferolateral extension) (Nikus et al. 2004). The ST elevation in V_{5-6} is explained by the presence of a local injury vector (see above) (Figure 28). However, in leads I and aVL ST-segment depression is seen, while in the case of a quite dominant LCX frequently there is ST depression

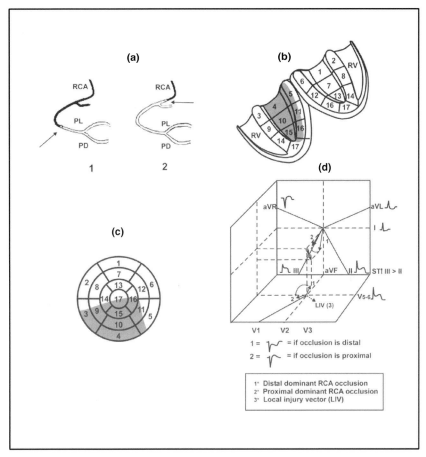

Figure 28 STEMI due to occlusion of a very dominant RCA: (a) site of occlusion may be before or after the RV branches; (b) myocardial area at risk; (c) polar map in "bull's-eye" projection with the most involved segments marked in gray; (d) injury vector is important and directed downward but may present a direction more or less to the right according to the placement of the occlusion before or after the RV branches (1: distal, 2: proximal). The projection of the injury vector in the different hemifields explains the ST morphology. However, the presence of ST elevation in V_{5-6} is explained by a local injury vector (LIV) (see text).

in aVL, usually in lead I, and ST may be slightly elevated, isodiphasic, and, only in rare cases, mildly depressed (Figures 34 and 35).

A typical electrocardiographic example of this type of STEMI is shown in Figure 29.

In the subacute and chronic phases the involvement of both lateral and inferior walls explains the Q wave in inferior leads and the RS morphology in V_1 because the necrosis vector of the inferolateral zone points to V_1 (see Figure 5).

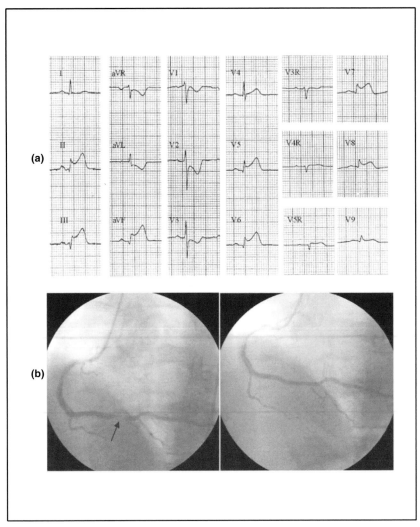

Figure 29 (a) The ECG in the case of a very dominant RCA occlusion distal to the RV branches. Observe that criteria of RCA occlusion are present: ST elevation in III is greater than that in II; ST elevation in the inferior leads is greater than ST depression in V_{1-3}, and furthermore ST elevation in V_{5-6} is greater than or equal to 2 mm. Note that in this case the first step of the algorithm of Figure 37 (ST depression in I) is not useful to diagnose RCA occlusion. The sum of ST deviations is higher than that seen in the case of a not very dominant RCA occlusion also distal to the RV branches (see Figure 27).

LCX occlusion proximal to the first OM branch

In this case (Figure 30a) the **area at risk** encompasses the majority of the lateral wall and may also compromise the inferior wall, especially the inferobasal segment. In Figure 30b and c the involved myocardial area along with the

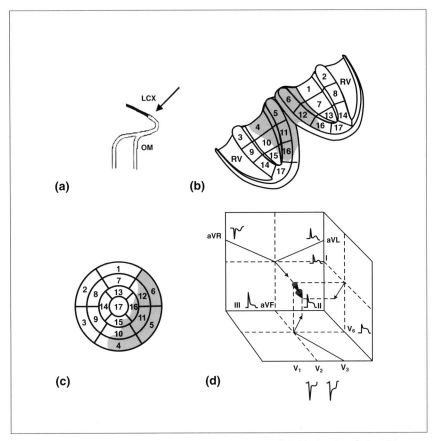

Figure 30 STEMI due to proximal occlusion of nondominant LCX: (a) site of occlusion; (b) myocardial area at risk; (c) polar map in "bull's-eye" projection with the most involved segments marked in gray; (d) injury vector is directed usually more backward than downward and to the left. Its projection in frontal, horizontal, and sagittal planes explains the corresponding ECG patterns, with ST depression in V_{1-3} often more evident than ST elevation in inferior leads and ST elevation in II greater than that in III (see text).

corresponding polar map in the case of balanced dominance are shown. The most affected segments are 4, 5, 6, 10, 11, and 12, and part of segment 16.

The **injury vector** is directed leftward and more posteriorly than downward. The projection of this vector in FP and HP explains (Figures 30d and 31) that the ST elevation in II is greater than or equal to that in III and that the ST-segment depression in V_{1-3} is of a higher voltage than the ST elevation in II, III, and aVF. Sometimes the difference in voltage is striking, with more than 5 mm of ST depression in the right precordial leads and only 1–3 mm of elevation in the inferior leads (see also Cases 1 and 15 in Chapter 6). This is probably related to the evidence that the inferobasal segment of the inferior

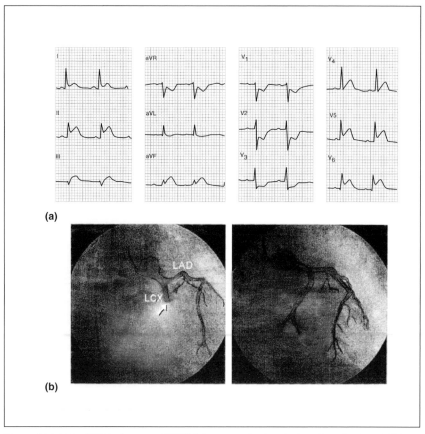

(a)

(b)

Figure 31 (a) The ECG in the case of STEMI due to proximal occlusion of nondominant LCX. Observe ST elevation in II, III, VF (II > III) and in I and V_6, and ST depression in V_{1-3} is greater than ST elevation in the inferior leads. (b) Coronary angiography before (left) and after (right) reperfusion. The arrow indicates the place of occlusion.

wall of the heart, usually perfused by a nondominant LCX, clearly bends upward. However, in spite of that, these are cases of STEMI that may benefit from reperfusion therapy (see Case 1 in Chapter 6).

A typical example of this type of STEMI is shown in Figure 31a, along with its correlation with the coronary angiogram (Figure 31b) before and after fibrinolytic therapy.

Occlusion of the first OM branch

When the occlusion is located in the first OM branch from the LCX (Figure 32a), the **area at risk** includes a great portion of the anterior and also the posterior part of the lateral wall (Figure 32b and c). The OM takes off from the LCX in the left ventricular obtuse margin and, after perfusing the basal lateral wall (anterior and posterior parts), is directed downward along the border of the

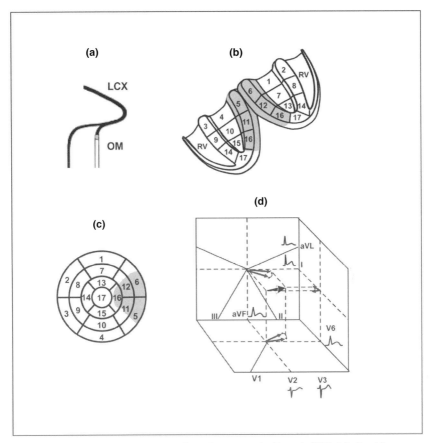

Figure 32 STEMI due to the occlusion of the obtuse marginal branch (OM): (a) site of the occlusion; (b) myocardial area at risk; (c) polar map of the affected area; (d) injury vector that is directed to the left and somewhat posteriorly, and usually upward, in the limit of positive hemifield of aVF and V_2, but sometimes downward and backward. Occasionally, if it is small, it hardly produces any ST changes. If they occur, ST-segment elevation is observed in the leads facing the lateral wall and/or the inferior leads especially II and aVF. V_{1-3} usually show slight ST-segment depression. In the case of a STEMI secondary to the selective occlusion of D_1, in V_{2-3} usually ST-segment elevation is observed (Figure 21), but especially in the presence of two/three-vessel disease mild ST-segment depression may be seen (see Case 9 in Chapter 6).

lateral wall, often reaching the low portion of that wall. The most involved area is part of segments 5, 6, 12, and 16. The perfusion of this area is shared with a ramus intermedius when present.

The **injury vector** is directed to the left and somewhat posteriorly, as well as somewhat upward or downward (Figure 32d). The projection of this vector in the positive and negative hemifields of different leads of the FP and HP explains the slight ST-segment elevation that is usually seen in the so-called lateral wall leads (I, aVL, V_{5-6}) and sometimes also in the inferior leads, especially II and aVF (Figure 33). On occasion the injury vector is directed more downward and

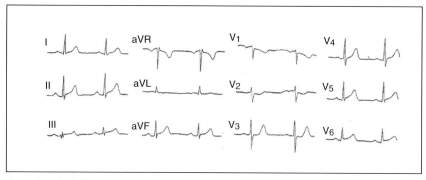

Figure 33 The ECG in the case of STEMI due to occlusion of obtuse marginal artery (OM). Observe slight ST elevation in I, II, III, VF, and V_{5-6}, with a slight depression in V_{1-3} (compare with Figure 20).

in this case the ST is elevated in the inferior leads and may be depressed in aVL (see Case 13 in Chapter 6). Since the injury vector is directed somewhat posteriorly, slight ST-segment depression may be seen from V_1 to V_3 (Figure 33), rather than ST-segment elevation that is frequently seen (usually from V_2 to V_4) in the STEMI due to the first diagonal branch occlusion (Figures 20 and 21). This is because the injury vector in the first diagonal occlusion is also directed leftward, but upward and somewhat anteriorly. In the occlusion of the first OM it is usually directed also to the left, but somewhat posteriorly and usually a little downwards (Birnbaum et al. 1996) (compare Figures 20d and 32d). When the OM branch is small, the changes can be minimal, if they do occur. In fact, the ECG often is normal.

In the subacute or chronic phase, "QR" or "R" morphology in "lateral leads" (I, aVL, and/or V_{5-6}) may be present frequently with RS (R) in V_1, but never QS in aVL. On the contrary, in STEMI due to the first diagonal occlusion, QS morphology in aVL may be present but without Q wave in V_{5-6}.

A typical example of this STEMI is shown in Figure 33, which in this case did not evolve to a Q-wave infarction in the chronic phase (normal ECG).

Occlusion of a very dominant LCX
When the LCX is very dominant (Figure 34a) and the occlusion is proximal, the **area at risk** involves a great part of the inferolateral zone that includes the majority of the lateral and inferior walls and even some portion of the posterior part of the septum. The involved segments are 3, 4, 5, 6, 9, 10, 11, 12, 15, and 16 (Figure 34b and c).

The **injury vector** in the case of a very dominant LCX is important and less directed to the left. The injury vector is located often in the FP between +60° and +90°. This means that it may fall in the negative hemifield of aVL but is usually still in the positive hemifield of lead I or in the limit of two hemifields. This explains (Figure 34d) why there may be often a small amount of ST-segment depression in lead aVL and an isodiphasic pattern or even in rare cases a small

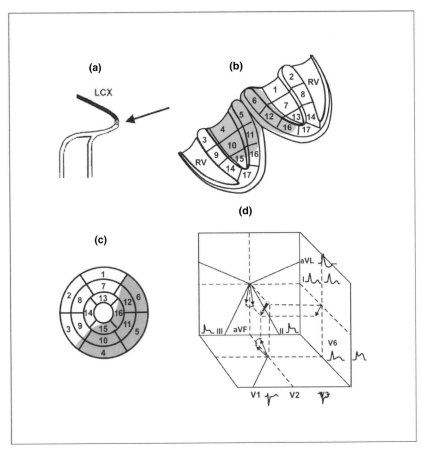

Figure 34 STEMI due to proximal occlusion of very dominant LCX: (a) site of occlusion; (b) myocardial area at risk; (c) polar map in "bull's-eye" projection with the most involved segments marked in gray; (d) injury vector is important and directed more backward than downward and less to the left or even a little to the right as projected in frontal, horizontal, and sagittal planes, with corresponding ECG patterns of ST depression and elevation (see text).

depression in lead I (see Case 15 in Chapter 6). The ST-segment elevation in II, III, and VF is often smaller than the ST depression in V_{1-3}. In the case that the ST elevation in II, III, and VF is equal or superior to ST depression in V_{1-3}, usually the ST elevation in II is greater than that in III and in lead I there is no clear ST depression as usually happens in the case of the proximal occlusion of a very dominant RCA. Also, the ST elevation in V_{5-6} in the occlusion of a very dominant LCX is usually more evident than in a case of a very dominant RCA (see Figures 29 and 35).

In the case of distal occlusion of a very dominant LCX the ECG characteristics are very similar to those in the case of distal occlusion of a short RCA.

A typical electrocardiographic example of this type of STEMI is shown in Figure 35.

2. From the electrocardiographic pattern to the occluded artery and the area at risk

From a clinical standpoint, one could state that in the majority of cases the most striking ECG abnormality found by the practitioner is ST-segment elevation in the precordial leads (V_{1-6}) (anteroseptal zone) (Figure 36) or in the inferior leads (inferolateral zone) (Figure 37). We will see that based on these data, one could identify not only the culprit artery but also the occlusion site (Fiol et al. 2004a–c).

Most striking ST-segment elevation in the precordial leads (V_{1-2} to V_{4-6})

The most striking ST-segment elevation is seen in the precordial leads (V_{1-2} to V_{4-6}). This corresponds to an LAD occlusion (Bayés de Luna & Fiol 2006, Engelen et al. 1999, Haraphongse et al. 1984, Porter et al. 1998, Sapin et al. 1992, Tamura et al. 1995).

The rationale to follow in order to determine the characteristics of the occluded artery and the site of occlusion is shown in Figure 36.

Firstly, the ST-segment should be assessed (to check for the presence or absence of depression) in II, III, and VF, and also its deviations in aVR, V_1, and V_6 (see Figures 9 and 11). According to the ST-segment changes, the occlusion may be localized as proximal or distal to the first diagonal (D_1) and/or first septal (S_1) branch.

a When the ST-segment in II, III, and aVF is depressed (≥ 2.5 mm in III + aVF), the occlusion is probably proximal to the first diagonal (D_1) or to the second diagonal (D_2) if the first diagonal is very small. When the ST-segment is also elevated in V_1 and/or aVR or depressed in V_6 (ST ↑ in V_1 and aVR + ST ↓ in $V_6 > 0$), the occlusion is probably also proximal to the first septal (S_1). When this sum is less than 0, the occlusion probably is between S_1 and D_1. STEMI of similar ECG characteristics may be seen in cases of ischemia due to multiple-vessel disease (see p. 52). Even cases with involvement of the left main trunk, that usually present as huge ST depression, may show STEMI if there is no previous ischemia (no collateral circulation) as happens in coronary dissection.

b When the ST-segment is isoelectric (between <0.5-mm elevation of ST and <0.5-mm depression of ST) or shows elevation in II, III, and VF, the occlusion is distal to D_1. Then, leads aVR, V_1, and/or V_6 should be assessed to ascertain whether the occlusion is also distal to S_1 (ST ↑ in aVR and V_1 + ST ↓ in $V_6 < 0$), which occurs most frequently. In the infrequent cases that S_1 takes off after the D_1 branch and the occlusion is distal to D_1 but proximal to S_1, the ST is isodiphasic or elevated in the inferior leads (distal to D_1) and the sum of ST elevation in aVR and V_1 and ST depression in V_6 is greater than 0 (proximal to S_1). In these rare cases the inferior lead with the most evident ST elevation is lead III (III > II) because the injury vector in this case is directed downward and rightward and from lead III its head is better seen

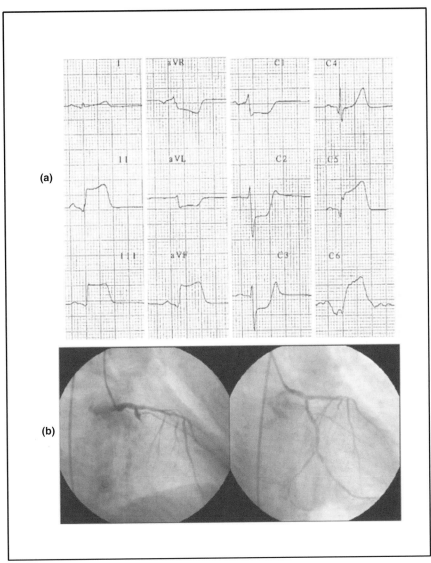

Figure 35 The ECG in the case of STEMI due to proximal occlusion of a very dominant LCX artery. Observe the criteria of LCX occlusion. ST elevation in II is greater than in III in the presence of isoelectric ST in I (second step of the algorithm of Figure 37). In aVL there is ST depression due to LCX dominance. In the normal cases of LCX occlusion there is no ST depression in VL (isoelectric or elevated) (Figure 31). Also a large ST elevation in V_{5-6} is more evident than in the case of very dominant RCA (Figure 29). On the other hand, the sum of ST deviations is much higher than in the case of proximal occlusion of a nondominant LCX (Figure 31).

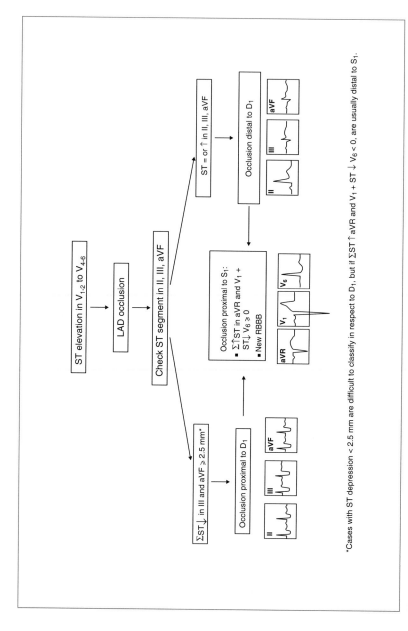

Figure 36 The algorithm to localize the site of LAD occlusion in the case of STEMI with predominant ST elevation in the precordial leads (see text).

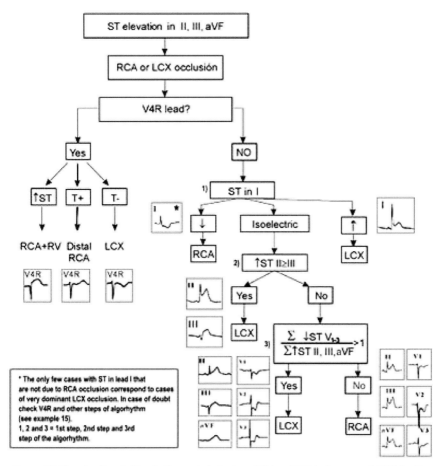

Figure 37 The algorithm to identify the occluded artery (RCA vs LCX) in the case of STEMI with ST elevation in the inferior leads (see text).

because the vector fails more in the positive hemifield of this lead (Figure 19). On the contrary, when the occlusion is distal to S_1 and D_1, ST elevation in II is greater than in III because the injury vector is directed to the apex (see Figure 17).

c **When the ST-segment is only slightly depressed** (<2.5 mm in III + VF), it is harder to classify with respect to D_1, but if "the septal branches involvement formula" (ST ↑ in aVR and V_1 + ST ↓ in V_6) is less than or equal to 0, the occlusion is probably distal to S_1 and D_1.

We have demonstrated (Fiol 2006) that STEMI due to the LAD occlusion proximal to S_1 and D_1 has, compared with other types of LAD STEMI, a higher Killip class in the acute phase and a lower final left ejection fraction in the chronic phase ($p < 0.05$).

Additionally, when a **typical right bundle branch block pattern** is seen in the course of a STEMI, it strongly suggests high septal ischemia (occlusion above the S_1 branch) as the cause of this conduction abnormality, since the S_1 branch perfuses the right bundle branch (see Case 7 in Chapter 6). This sign is very specific (100%) but not sensitive (14%) according to Gorgels et al. (2003).

Most striking ST-segment elevation recorded in II, III, and VF, or ST depression in V_{1-3}

The most striking ST-segment elevation is recorded in II, III, and VF, or ST depression in V_{1-3} as a mirror image, when the inferobasal–lateral segments are preferentially involved. **This corresponds to an RCA or LCX occlusion** (Figure 37) (Birnbaum et al. 1994; , Fiol et al. 2004c, Herz et al. 1997; Kosuge et al. 1998; Lew et al. 1986; Saw et al. 2001; Tamura et al. 1995).

In these cases it may be useful to assess the ST/T in V_4R to know whether the occlusion is located in the proximal or distal RCA or in the LCX (Figure 37) (Wellens et al. 2003). Since V_4R is sometimes not recorded and because abnormalities occurring in this lead are often quite transient, **we use a sequential approach based on the ST changes seen in the 12-lead surface ECG in order to ascertain whether the RCA or the LCX is the culprit artery** (Figure 37) (Fiol et al. 2004c).

a **First step: Assess the ST-segment in lead I.** In the case of depression, the occlusion is located in the RCA; in the case of elevation, it is located in the LCX. **When the ST-segment is isoelectric, one should proceed to the second step.**

b **Second step: Check the ST-segment in II, III, and VF.** When the ST elevation in II is greater than or equal to that in III, the occlusion is located in the LCX. **When the ST elevation in III is greater than or equal to that in II, one should proceed to the third step.**

c **Third step: The following relation should be assessed**

$$\frac{\sum ST \downarrow \text{ in } V_{1-3}}{\sum ST \uparrow \text{ in II, III, and VF}}$$

When the ratio is greater than 1, the culprit artery is the LCX; when it is equal to or less than 1, the culprit artery is the RCA.

With this sequential approach one may distinguish whether the RCA or the LCX is the culprit artery in over 95% of cases (Fiol et al. 2004c).

Once the RCA has been accurately determined to be the culprit artery, **it is important to know whether the occlusion is proximal or distal.** For that determination, **lead V_1** is important, and to a lesser degree leads I and aVL. Generally, an isoelectric or elevated ST-segment is seen in V_1 in the proximal occlusion (Figure 38). This change may persist up to V_{3-4}, but usually the ST elevation in V_1 is greater than that in V_{3-4}. **In the distal LAD** occlusion, as has already been said, **ST-segment elevation may also be seen in the precordial and inferior leads.** However, in this case (a) the ST elevation in the precordial leads is usually much greater than that in the inferior leads; and (b) the ST

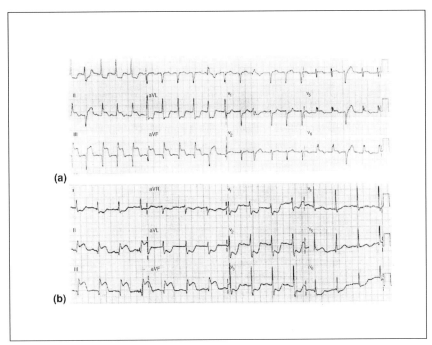

Figure 38 (a) The ECG in STEMI due to proximal RCA occlusion. ST depression in I and aVL (aVL > I) as well as ST in I and III (III > II) points to RCA occlusion, while the absence of ST depression in V_1 is an accurate criterion of right ventricular involvement (proximal occlusion), since in this case the injury vector points forward and rightward. As the RCA is dominant there is also ST elevation in V_{5-6} (local injury vector in Figure 28). (b) The ECG in STEMI due to distal RCA occlusion. In this case, the ST segment in the lateral and inferior leads shows similar behavior than in part (a) (RCA occlusion), but ST depression in V_{1-3} indicates distal occlusion, since the injury vector points backward (to the inferolateral wall) and as the RCA is not very dominant in V_6 there is no ST elevation.

elevation in V_{3-4} is greater than that in V_1. Furthermore, another ECG criterion in favor of RCA is the presence of ST-segment depression in lead I and aVL frequently less than 5 mm and in the case of distal LAD occlusion there is usually no clear ST depression in I and VL (Figures 17 and 25, Table 2).

If we compare the ECG patterns in the case of a very dominant RCA and LCX (Figures 29 and 35), we may see that both present with ST elevation in V_{5-6} and usually ST depression in aVL and sometimes an isoelectric ST segment in I but the presence of ST depression in lead I is much more in favor of RCA occlusion, although there are some exceptions (see Case 15 in Chapter 6). On the other hand, the presence of ST elevation in II greater than in III favors the LCX occlusion and vice versa (Figures 35a and 29a), and usually never in the case of very dominant RCA is the ST elevation in V_6 greater than 3–4 mm, as may happen in the case of a very dominant LCX (see Figure 35a).

ST elevation in inferior and precordial leads

This may be seen in STEMI due to occlusion of the distal LAD and very proximal RCA. The ECG criteria that support the occlusion in one or another artery are shown in Table 2, Figures 17 and 25, and Case 12 in Chapter 6.

The most striking ST-segment elevation in the lateral wall leads, I, aVL, and V_{5-6}

This may be seen in STEMI due to the **first–second diagonal occlusion** (or the LAD occlusion, involving the diagonal but not the septal branches), or the **first–second OM or, occasionally, the ramus intermedius branch occlusion**.

The diagnosis of a **first diagonal branch occlusion or equivalent** is favored by the presence of more significant ST-segment elevation in the so-called lateral wall leads (V_6, I, and aVL) than in the inferior leads (in which ST depression is usually seen) (Figure 21). Instead, in an **OM occlusion**, slight ST elevation may be seen in both groups of leads, since the injury vector is not upwardly directed (compare Figures 21 and 33) and even may be directed downward, in which case ST elevation may be seen only in the inferior leads (see Case 13 in Chapter 6). Generally, ST-segment elevation evident in the precordial leads (from V_{2-3} to V_{5-6}) may be seen in a first diagonal branch occlusion. This is explained by the direction of the injury vector, which usually points somewhat anteriorly. However, in some rare occasions, usually in the presence of multiple-vessel occlusion (D_1 + LCX or RCA) we have seen slight ST depression in V_{2-3} in STEMI due to the D_1 occlusion. On the contrary, ST-segment elevation in the precordial leads is not present in STEMI due to the OM branch occlusion. In this case slight ST-segment depression or just minimal ECG changes are seen, since the OM occlusion usually generates an injury vector that is directed somewhat posteriorly (compare Figures 21 and 33). In some cases, these STEMI's may hardly cause any ECG change.

In the chronic phase the limited anterolateral infarction due to a **first diagonal occlusion** may cause a QS morphology in aVL and even in lead I. However, no Q wave is seen in V_{5-6}. On the contrary, in the infarction secondary to the **OM branch occlusion**, a "QR" morphology may be seen in V_{5-6} and even in I and aVL, or merely a low-voltage R wave, but in general no QS morphology in aVL.

Sometimes involvement of the lateral wall is seen in the STEMI of both the anteroseptal zone (due to the LAD occlusion proximal to the diagonal branches, Figures 14 and 21) and the inferolateral zone (secondary to an occlusion of the LCX [I, VL, and/or V_{5-6}, Figures 31 and 35] or a dominant RCA [only V_{5-6}, Figure 29]). When the RCA is very dominant, the ST-segment elevation in V_{5-6} is usually greater than or equal to 2 mm (Nikus et al. 2005) but in cases of very dominant LCX the ST elevation in V_{5-6} may be even bigger (Figure 35).

ST deviations in aVR and additional leads

Due to occlusion of the LAD, ST deviation may also be seen in an aVR in some cases of STEMI. This occurs when the occlusion is proximal to S_1. However, in these cases there are ST elevations that are more striking in other leads (Figures 13 and 19).

On the other hand, the presence of ST elevation greater than or equal to 0.5 mm in aVR in NSTEMI with often very significant ST depression in many leads ($\geq$8) favors the diagnosis of incomplete occlusion of left main trunk or three-vessel disease. In the case of left main trunk involvement the ST depression usually is large and there is no final positive T wave in V_{4-5} (Kosuge et al. 2005, Yamaji et al. 2001). In some cases also with ST depression in many leads but with more evident ST depression in precordial than FP leads and with final positive T wave in V_{4-5}, the occlusion is in the proximal LAD (Bayés de Luna & Fiol 2006; Nikus et al. 2005).

We have already explained that the morphology of V_4R has been considered useful to discern the place of occlusion in RCA or LCX (see Figure 37 and page 48). However V_4R is not frequently recorded and abnormalities in that lead usually appear transiently in the hyperacute phase. A useful surrogate for V_4R is V_1 (Fiol et al. 2004a). However, if V_4R is recorded, it is useful to check the concordance with the morphology of V_1 so as to recognize the place of occlusion, although sometimes there is some discrepancy between the morphology of V_1 and V_4R (see Case 14 in Chapter 6).

Lastly, posterior leads may also be useful, although they are not often recorded. It has been considered that the use of additional extreme right precordial and posterior leads only slightly increases the diagnostic sensitivity obtained with the classical 12-lead surface ECG (Schmitt et al. 2001, Zalenski et al. 1997).

The algorithms presented in Figures 36 and 37, and other ST changes in lateral leads, aVR, and also additional leads, help us to accurately locate the place of the occlusion and consequently to know the importance of the area at risk. Tables 3 and 4 show the most important ECG criteria related to the site of coronary occlusion (see pp. 57–58).

Other characteristics of ST elevation regarding prognosis

Quantification of the area at risk by the summation of the ST-segment elevations and depressions

In order to quantify the area at risk, both ST-segment elevations and depressions should be assessed. The latter are not the expression of subendocardial injury but the expression of subepicardial (transmural) injury in a distant area. Therefore, in LAD occlusion, ST depression detected in II, III, and VF, more significant when compared to ST elevation in the same leads, represents more ischemia (compare Figures 15 and 17). **The prognosis has been shown to**

be worse (higher possibilities of developing primary ventricular fibrillation) **when the summation of ST-segment deviations is significant (more than 15 mm) (Hathaway et al. 1998). Furthermore, the finding of ST-segment elevation greater than 8 mm in the three most compromised leads**, along with the presence of hypotension, is a marker of the poorest prognosis, especially in cases with inferior infarction (Fiol et al. 1993).

However, some limitations may occur, e.g., in the case of infarction due to occlusion of a dominant RCA proximal to the RV branches. In spite of the large area involved, the ST-segment is frequently isoelectric or may even present as elevation in the right precordial leads, since the RV involvement counteracted the ST depression that is usually seen in the large infarctions due to the RCA occlusion. For this reason, the injury vector is directed more rightward (Figure 24) and masks the ST-segment depression in V_{1-3} (Figure 25). Therefore, at the same dominance of RCA, an occlusion before the RV branches (Figure 25) may be present; if the ST is isoelectric in V_{1-2}, fewer ST-segment changes than in an RCA occlusion after the take-off of the RV branch may be present (Figure 27).

Usefulness of ST morphology with regards to prognosis

Three ST/T elevation morphologies that could help in prognostication have been described (Figure 39) (Birnbaum et al. 1993). In cases with just slight ECG changes (tall and wide T wave; type A or grade 1), the prognosis is better than when the ST-segment is convex with respect to the isoelectric baseline (type B or grade 2) or, especially, when it is concave with distortion of the final portion of the QRS complex (type C or grade 3). In the latter case, the coronary occlusion probably is very proximal and not much collateral circulation exists. **The type C morphology usually presents with a ratio J point/R wave of greater than 0.5 (Figure 39c)**. This morphology expresses the involvement of the Purkinje fibers, which are more resistant to ischemia than are the myocytes. Therefore, it suggests that the area with acute ischemia is probably larger and more severe. Type C patterns may appear shortly after an episode of severe acute ischemia. These electrocardiographic findings are of great importance because they express the need for urgent treatment to avoid the progression of evolving myocardial infarction. It is especially important if the chest pain duration is similar in the different groups when the patients arrive at the hospital. When a patient arrives at the emergency room after 6 hours of chest pain with a normal ECG tracing (type A), the prognosis is better than if a normal ECG is recorded just 15 minutes from the onset of pain.

ST changes in patients with ischemia due to multivessel occlusion

All the cases of STEMI that have been discussed are due to ischemia generated by occlusion in one culprit vessel, though occlusions may be present in more than one vessel.

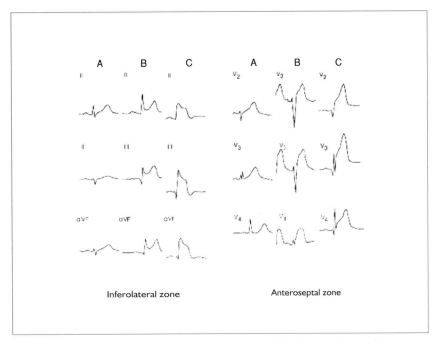

Figure 39 Observe the three types of repolarization abnormalities that may be seen in an acute phase of STEMI involving the inferolateral (left) and anteroseptal zones (right). (A) Tall and/or wide T waves especially present in STEMI of the anteroseptal zone. (B) Abnormal ST elevation, with no changes of the final part of QRS. (C) Important ST elevation and distortion of the final part of QRS (see text).

Although there are no clear electrocardiographic criteria, the following clues should alert clinicians that the ECG patterns may be explained by the critical involvement of two or more vessels:

1 In a patient with STEMI with ST elevation in II, III, and VF, the presence of ST depression in precordial leads beyond V_{2-3} with maximal changes in V_{4-5} may be explained by the occlusion of the RCA, plus a significant obstruction in the LAD (Nikus et al. 2005).

2 The presence of ST-segment elevation in the right precordial leads (V_{1-3}) and ST depression in the left-sided leads (aVL, I, V_{4-6}) suggests multivessel involvement (Kurum et al. 2002). In the STEMI due to the LAD occlusion proximal to D_1 and S_1 (single vessel disease), ST-segment elevation may also be recorded from V_1 to V_4 and ST depression in V_{5-6}. However, in the case of occlusion proximal to D_1 and S_1 the ST-segment depression is not seen in lead I; and in aVL if it exists the depression is mild (see Figures 12 and 13).

3 It has been shown that in a STEMI due to occlusion of long LAD distal to D_1 and S_1 the ST elevation originates in precordial leads and in II, III, and VF. However, this morphology may also be explained by an occlusion of the LAD in the presence of a total RCA occlusion with collateral vessels from

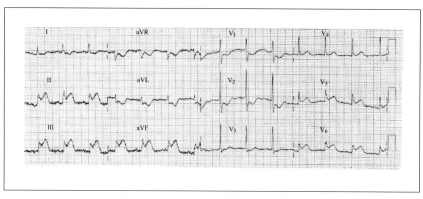

Figure 40 The ECG in STEMI due to very dominant RCA occclusion distal to the RV branches. ST depression in I points toward RCA occlusion. The ST elevation in III is greater than that in II and the ratio of ST depression in V_{1-3}/ST elevation in II, III, aVF less than 1 also favors RCA involvement. ST elevation in V_{5-6} suggests that the RCA is large enough to reach the low-inferolateral wall (superdominance). Coronary angiography showed not only very dominant RCA occlusion but also multiple but not critical LAD occlusions. Accurate interpretation of the ECG assures that the culprit artery is RCA and therefore a PCI was performed in this artery.

the LAD to the RCA, even in the absence of a considerably long LAD. There is not any ECG criterion that may help us to differentiate these two cases, because in both situations the ST elevation in the precordial leads is more important than that in the inferior leads.

4 The presence of slight ST depression in V_{2-4} in STEMI due to D_1 occlusion (ST elevation in I, aVL, V_{5-6} and ST depression in II, III, VF) suggests the presence of multiple-vessel disease, especially D_1 + LCX or RCA.

When a STEMI occurs a patient typically has a critical occlusion in only one culprit artery. In most cases, because multivessel disease is often present, what is most important is that in the catheterization laboratory, in a patient with STEMI and multiple-vessel disease, the interventional cardiologist makes the correct decision as to the coronary artery on which PCI is to be performed, thanks to the correct interpretation of the ECG (Figure 40). With the angiograhic results at hand, the ECG gives important information that helps in identifying the culprit artery in cases of multivessel disease, and unfortunately this information is largely underused in clinical decision making (Nikus et al. 2004, 2005). Therefore a closer collaboration among clinicians, experts in ECG, and interventionalists should be emphasized. This may be possible with modern technology that may give us an expert opinion at any distance even within seconds (Leibrand et al. 2000).

CHAPTER 5

Conclusions

This book emphasizes the importance of evaluation of the pattern of ST-segment deviation in patients with a narrow QRS and ST elevation-myocardial infarction (STEMI). This information allows clinicians to ascertain where the occlusion is located and identify the area of the left ventricle at risk. The deductive diagnostic approach described in this book (Figures 36 and 37 and Table 1) allows clinicians to locate the site of occlusion promptly after scrutinizing the 12-lead ECG. This is extremely important for not only correctly diagnosing a patient in urgent need of reperfusion but also defining the culprit artery if a percutaneous coronary intervention (PCI) is performed. Correct diagnosis of the culprit coronary artery is critical when considering PCI in a STEMI patient with multivessel disease. Tables 3 and 4 summarize the ST changes in STEMI due to occlusion of the different coronary arteries at different places. Table 5 shows the cases of STEMI that are at higher risk on admission and consequently need to be treated with more urgency.

It is our belief that, even with the limitations already expressed on page 15 and in Table 5, by applying the principles outlined in this book clinicians will be better informed about the prognosis of STEMI patients whose ECG has been recorded, and more effectively formulate the optimum approach for reperfusion therapy in a variety of clinical settings.

Table 3 STEMI: the ST-segment elevation in the precordial leads.

ECG criteria (ST deviations) supporting the place of occlusion LAD

1 **Occlusion of LAD above the D_1 branch:** ST elevation in V_2 to V_{4-6}. ST-segment depression is recorded in at least two inferior leads (III + aVF $\geq$ 2.5 mm), which in general is less important than the ST-segment elevation seen in the precordial leads.
2 **Occlusion of LAD below the D_1 branch:** ST elevation also in V_2 to V_{4-6}. No ST-segment depression is seen in II, III, and aVF. In turn, an isoelectric or not significantly elevated ST-segment is recorded in these leads.
3 **Occlusion of LAD above the S_1 branch:** Regardless of where D_1 is, there is ST-segment elevation in aVR and V_1 and ST-segment depression in V_6 because the injury vector is directed upward and rightward.
4 **Occlusion of LAD is located below the S_1 and D_1 branches:** ST elevation in V_2 to V_{4-6}. A generally slight ST-segment elevation is seen in leads II, III, and aVF and there is no ST elevation in aVR and V_1.
5 **Occlusion of LAD involving septal but not diagonal branches or selective occlusion of S_1:** ST elevation in V_{1-2} and aVR and ST depression in II and V_6.
6 **Occlusion of LAD involving diagonal but not septal branches or selective occlusion of D_1:** Often ST elevation in I, aVL, V_{5-6}, and sometimes even in more precordial leads, and ST depression in II, III, and aVF.

Table 4 STEMI: ST elevation in inferior and lateral leads.

ECG criteria (ST-deviations) supporting an occlusion of the RCA, LCX, D$_1$, and OM

1 Occlusion of the RCA

   a There is usually ST-segment depression in I and aVL. In general, ST-segment depression in aVL is greater than in I.

   b The ST-segment elevation in III is usually greater than that in II.

   c The ST-segment depression in the right precordial leads is usually smaller than the ST-segment elevation in the inferior leads. This is especially true when the occlusion is proximal to the RV branches, in which case the ST-segment in V$_{3-4}$ is usually isoelectric or even elevated but with ST elevation in V$_1$ greater than in V$_{3-4}$. On the contrary, in the cases of LAD occlusion ST elevation in V$_{3-4}$ is greater than in V$_1$.

   d When the RCA is dominant, ST-segment elevation is seen in V$_5$ and V$_6$. ST-segment elevation $\geq$ 2 mm in these leads indicates that the RCA is very dominant.

2 Occlusion of the LCX proximal to first OM branch

   a There is usually ST elevation in I and aVL.

   b The ST-segment elevation in II is usually equal to or greater than that in III.

   c The ST-segment elevation in II, III, and aVF is usually smaller than the ST depression in the right precordial leads. Sometimes this is quite apparent.

   d When the LCX is quite dominant it may present the above-mentioned criteria but often with evident ST depression in aVL, but very rarely in I.

3 Occlusion of the OM

   a There is usually ST-segment elevation in the so-called lateral leads, I, aVL, and V$_{5-6}$. Sometimes this change is only present in the inferior leads, especially II and aVF.

   b There is often slight ST depression in V$_{1-3}$.

4 Occlusion of the D$_1$

   a ST-segment elevation may be seen in the so-called "lateral wall" leads, especially in I and aVL. In fact, these leads face the anterior and often the mid-low lateral wall, but not the high lateral wall. Since the injury vector is directed more upward and, generally, anteriorly with regards to what occurs in an OM occlusion, ST-segment depression is usually recorded in the inferior leads.

   b ST-segment elevation may be seen in the precordial leads, sometimes as from V$_2$ to V$_3$ and occasionally with evident elevation. In turn, the ST-segment in V$_{2-3}$ is usually isoelectric or depressed in the OM occlusion (compare Figures 21 and 33). Rarely in the case of D$_1$ occlusion slight ST depression may be seen in the precordial leads. This usually represents multiple-vessel occlusion (D$_1$ + LCX or RCA especially).

Table 5 STEMI: prognostic value of the ST-segment deviations on admission.

1 **Check the location of ST-segment elevation or depression**
   The cases at higher risk are those caused by:
   a **Proximal LAD occlusion (especially proximal to S_1 and D_1). This includes the presence of some of the following criteria:**
      - ST elevation in V_1 to V_5
      - Clear ST-segment depression in II, III, aVF, and V_6 and ST elevation in aVR, aVL, and I
      - New right bundle branch block and, sometimes, left bundle branch block or bifascicular block
   b **A very dominant RCA occlusion (especially when the obstruction is proximal to the RV branches). This includes:**
      - ST elevation in II, III, VF (III > II)
      - ST elevation in V_6 ≥ 2 mm
      - ST isoelectric or positive in VI in the case of proximal occlusion of RCA
   c **A very dominant LCX occlusion.**
      - Important ST elevation in II, III, VF (II $\geq$ III) that often is greater than ST depression in V_{1-3}
      - ST elevation in left precordial leads sometimes is very large ($\geq$ 4–5 mm)
      - Often in the case of very dominant LCX occlusion, the segment ST is depressed in aVL but rarely in I. In the case of very dominant RCA, there is ST depression in I and aVL
2 **Check the sum in millimeters of the ST-segment elevations and depressions.**
   - Figures above 15 mm usually represent a large area at risk
   - There are some limitations. In the case of RV involvement, the ST in V_{1-2} is often isoelectric and in spite of high risk that the RV involvement represents, the lack of deviation of the ST segment in these leads diminishes the sum of ST deviations.
3 **Check the ST-segment morphology.**
   - Cases with the poorest prognosis are those presenting with concave ST-segment with regards to the isoelectric baseline, with distortion of the final portion of the QRS segment and ratio J point/R wave > 0.5

CHAPTER 6

Self-assessment

This section of the book gives the reader the opportunity to apply the principles of analysis of the pattern of ST-segment deviation in a series of 15 cases. Each case contains one or more 12-lead ECGs to be analyzed in a self-assessment fashion. The correct answer is to be selected from a multiple-choice list. A brief explanation of the correct answer follows along with the pivotal images from the coronary arteriogram demonstrating the point of occlusion and the culprit coronary artery. Cross-reference is made to the relevant polar maps and injury vector diagrams seen in the earlier parts of the book. The location of the occlusion along with other characteristics of the ECG and the clinical status of the patient will give the information necessary to take the final decision on the management of each case.

Case 1

Clinical background

A 52-year-old man is presented with clinical characteristics of acute coronary syndrome (ACS). Initially, non-STEMI was considered as the most striking ST change was ST depression in V_{1-3}. However, the presence of mild ST elevation in II, III, and VF and also in V_{5-6} suggested a STEMI. There is also isodiphasic ST in I and small ST depression in aVL.

Which is the culprit artery of this ACS?

a Non-STEMI due to LAD subocclusion
b STEMI due to LCX proximal occlusion
c STEMI due to RCA occlusion

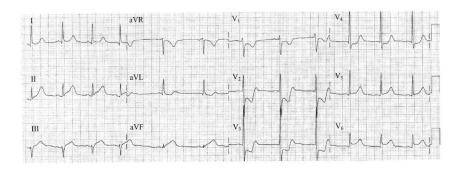

Answer to Case 1: b

The correct answer is **STEMI due to LCX proximal occlusion**.

We used the following logic:

1 Despite the most striking ST change being the ST depression in V_{1-3}, this is a STEMI, because there is mild ST elevation in II, III, aVF and in V_{5-6}. It is important that practitioners be aware that in the presence of this pattern, ST depression in V_{1-3} is a mirror image of ST elevation in the lateral–inferobasal wall.

2 This mirror image is usually due to occlusion of LCX that perfuses the lateral-inferobasal wall segment. The huge ST depression is because in this case most probably the area involved in the injury is a portion of the inferior lateral wall, an inferobasal segment of inferior wall, and perhaps a portion of the mid-inferior segment that bends upwards (see p. 5). Therefore, in the case of injury of this area, the injury vector faces V_{1-3} (see Figure 5).

3 The diagnosis of LCX occlusion is based on the algorithm in Figure 37: ST isodiphasic in I, ST II > III, but clearly ST ↓ $V_1 - V_3$/ST ↑ inferior leads > 1.

4 This pattern in V_{1-3} may also be seen in the case of non-proximal dominant RCA (see Figure 5), but in this case ST elevation in III > II, and ST ↓ $V_1 - V_3$/ST ↑ inferior leads < 1.

5 This case is similar to Case 15. However, the ST in lead I is isodiphasic and in Case 15 is mildly negative. The presence of ST depression in lead I (Case 15) is very rare even in the cases of proximal LCX occlusion. As a matter of fact, its presence favors the diagnosis of RCA occlusion (Figure 37). In these situations the ECG pattern of right precordial leads may be useful because the presence of negative T waves favors LCX occlusion (see Case 15). We have only seen ST depression when the LCX is very dominant and the occlusion is very proximal, because then the majority of the inferolateral territory is supplied by LCX. However, when the occlusion of very dominant LCX is very distal, the territory at risk is approximately the same as in the case of distal occlusion of short RCA and in both cases the ECG's are usually similar, and rarely abnormal.

(*continued on next page*)

Figure 30 shows how the projection of the injury vector on the FP and HP explains the ST morphology in different leads in the case of proximal occlusion of the LCX.

Pre-PCI   **Post-PCI**

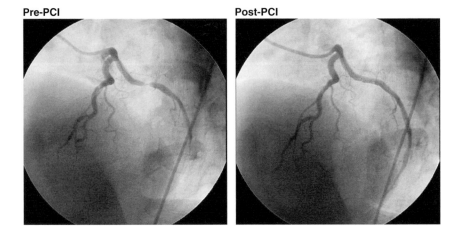

Case 2

Clinical background

A 48-year-old man presents with clinical characteristics compatible with a STEMI without hemodynamic compromise.

The ECG shows:

1 ST elevation in II, III, and aVF and slight ST elevation in V_{5-6} (<2 mm)
2 ST depression in V_{1-3}

Which is the culprit artery of this STEMI?

a Proximal dominant RCA
b Distal dominant RCA
c LCX

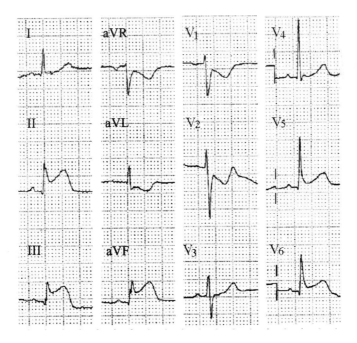

Answer to Case 2: b

The correct answer is a **distal dominant RCA but not superdominant** (see coronary angiography).

We used the following logic:

1 The first two steps of the algorithm in Figure 37 are not definitive: ST is isoelectric in I and ST elevation in III is similar to that in II. However, clearly the third step of the algorithm favors RCA occlusion (ST elevation in II, III, aVF is greater than ST depression in V_{1-3}). Therefore the culprit artery is RCA.

2 The occlusion is distal, because evident ST depression in V_{1-3} is present.

3 The RCA is dominant, but not superdominant, because the ST elevation in V_{5-6} is a little smaller than 2 mm (Eskola et al. 2004).

Figure 28 shows how the projection of the injury vector on the FP and HP explains the ST morphology in different leads in the case of proximal and distal occlusion of dominant RCA. In Figure 29 there is an example of distal occlusion of a superdominant RCA (ST elevation in $V_6 \geq 2$ mm).

Pre-PCI

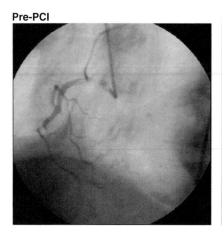

Post-PCI

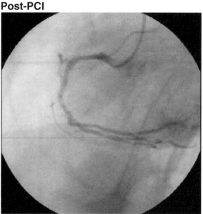

Case 3

Clinical background

A 57-year-old man is seen with clinical characteristics compatible with an ACS. The ECG shows:

1 ST depression in I and aVL (aVL > I)
2 ST elevation in II, III, and aVF (III > II)
3 ST depression in V_{1-3} but lesser than ST elevation in II, III, and aVF
4 ST flattened or slightly depressed in V_{5-6}

Which is the culprit artery of this STEMI?

a Proximal and dominant RCA
b Distal and short RCA
c LCX

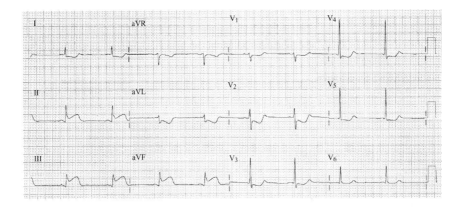

Answer to Case 3: b

The correct answer is **distal and short RCA**.

We used the following logic:

1 The ECG presents the three diagnostic steps from the algorithm presented in Figure 37, which indicates that the culprit artery is the RCA:

a ST depression in I

b ST elevation in III greater than in II

c ST elevation more important in the inferior wall than ST depression in V_{1-3}

2 The occlusion is *distal to the RV branches* because ST depression is present from V_1 to V_3. In general, from our experience, V_1 is at least as reliable as V_4R for the decision whether the occlusion is distal or proximal. Thus, it is usually enough to use V_1 in clinical practice (see Case 15).

3 Finally, the RCA is short, because no ST elevation is present in the left precordial leads. However, the occlusion is complete and this explains the fact that the burden of ischemia is large (the sum of ST depressions is greater than 15 mm).

Figure 26 shows how the projection of the injury vector on the FP and HP explains the ST morphology in different leads in the case of distal occlusion of a short RCA.

Pre-PCI   **Post-PCI**

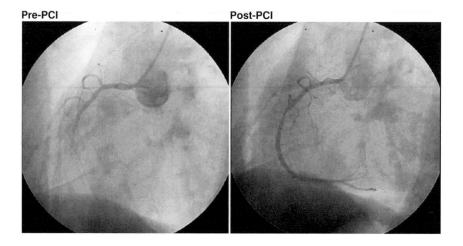

Case 4

Clinical background

A 57-year-old woman presents with acute chest pain of 2 hours duration with clinical characteristics of ACS.

The ECG shows:

1 ST-segment elevation from V_1 to V_4 and in aVR and mild elevation in aVL
2 ST-segment depression in II, III, aVF, and V_6

Which is the culprit artery of this STEMI?

a LAD proximal to D_1 and S_1
b LAD distal to S_1 and D_1
c LAD subocclusion encompassing diagonal branches but not septal branches (or selective D_1 occlusion)

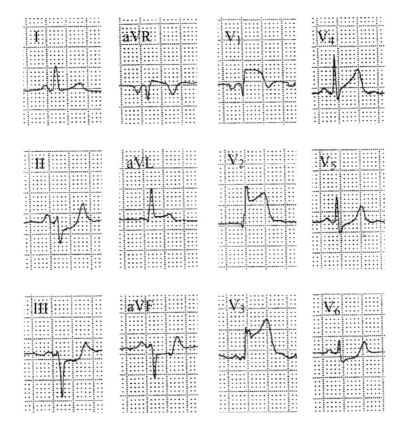

Answer to Case 4: a

The correct answer is **LAD occlusion proximal to D_1 and S_1**.

We used the following logic:

1 The presence of ST elevation in V_{1-4} with ST depression in III and VF greater than or equal to 2.5 mm strongly suggests LAD occlusion proximal to D_1.

2 The presence of $\Sigma ST\uparrow$ VR and $V_1 + ST\downarrow$ in $V_6 > 0$ suggests that the occlusion is also proximal to S_1.

3 In LAD occlusion proximal to D_1 and S_1 the $ST\downarrow$ in II is greater than in III (see page 12 and 13).

4 LAD occlusion distal to D_1 and S_1 would present isodiphasic or elevated ST in II, III, and VF.

5 LAD subocclusion encompassing septal but not diagonal branches may also cause ST depression in II, III, VF and $ST\uparrow$ VR and $V_1 + ST\downarrow$ in $V_6 > 0$, but usually the ST elevation is not so striking in V_{1-4} and in aVL there is no ST elevation (as in this case), because the injury vector is directed more to the right (see Figure 20).

Figure 12 shows how the projection of the injury vector on the FP and HP explains the ST morphology in different leads in the case of LAD occlusion proximal to S_1 and D_1 (see arrow).

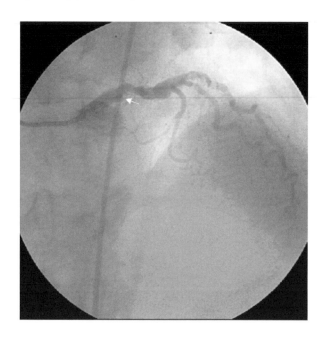

Case 5

Clinical background

A 62-year-old man presents with clinical characteristics compatible with an ACS.

The ECG presents the morphology of one STEMI with ST elevation in II, III, aVF, V_5, and V_6 and ST depression in I, aVL, and from V_1 to V_3.

Which is the culprit artery of this STEMI?
a Proximal occlusion of dominant RCA
b Nonproximal occlusion of very dominant RCA
c Proximal LCX

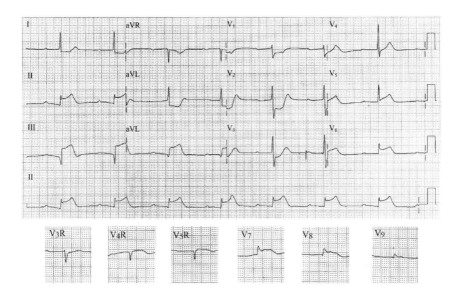

Answer to Case 5: b

The correct answer is **nonproximal occlusion of very dominant RCA** (see coronary angiography).

The logic we followed in this case was the following:

1 There is no doubt that the culprit artery is the RCA, because the ST-segment is depressed in I (first level of the algorithm presented in Figure 37). Additionally, the ST elevation in III is greater than that in II and ST depression in V_{1-3} is smaller than the ST elevation in II, III, and aVF.

2 It is nonproximal, because there is evident ST depression in V_{1-2}. In this case even in V_4R there is no clear elevation, which is in favor of a distal occlusion.

3 The RCA is very dominant because there is an ST elevation greater than or equal to 2 mm in V_6.

4 The occlusion is total and the area at risk is large (>30 mm of ST deviations).

Figure 28 shows how the projection of the injury vector on the FP and HP explains the ST morphology in different leads in the case of nonproximal occlusion of very dominant RCA (vector 1).

Pre-PCI   Post-PCI

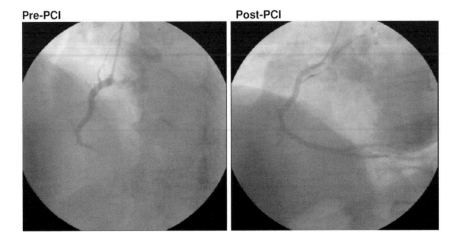

Case 6

Clinical background

A 67-year-old woman is seen with clinical characteristics of ACS. The ECG corresponds to a STEMI with ST elevation in precordial leads from V_1 to V_6 and also slight elevation in II and isoelectric ST in III and aVF. The ST is depressed in aVR.

Which is the culprit artery of this STEMI?

a LAD proximal to D_1 and S_1
b LAD distal to D_1 and S_1
c LAD proximal to D_1 and distal to S_1

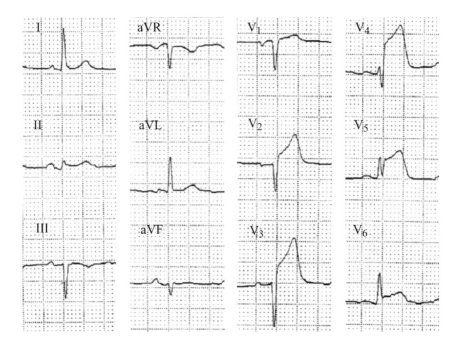

Answer to Case 6: b

The correct answer is **LAD distal to D_1 and S_1**.

We used the following logic.

It is clear that the occlusion is of the LAD (striking ST elevation in all precordial leads). In this case:

1 The fact that the ST-segment is isodiphasic or elevated in II, III, aVF strongly suggests that the occlusion is distal to D_1 (see Figure 36).

2 On the other hand the ST-segment is slightly elevated in V_1, but depressed in aVR and elevated in V_6 in a manner that ST↑ in V_1 and aVR + ST↓ in $V_6 < 0$. This supports the fact that the occlusion of the LAD is also distal to S_1.

3 The ECG patterns in V_4 and sum of ST deviations suggest that very acute and extensive ischemia exists. However, the fact that the location of occlusion is distal to S_1 and D_1 favors the likelihood that the area at risk is not as huge as suggested.

Figure 17 shows how the projection of the injury vector on the FP and HP explains the ST morphology in different leads in the case of LAD occlusion distal to D_1 and S_1.

Pre-PCI

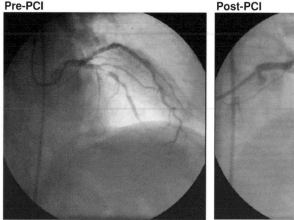

Post-PCI

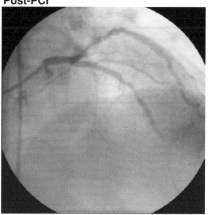

Case 7

Clinical background
A 47-year-old man presents with a clinical syndrome compatible with ACS of 3 hours duration. The ECG shows (Figure a) right bundle branch block (RBBB) with marked ST elevation in all precordial leads, I and aVL, and ST depression in II, III, and aVF. There is also ST elevation in aVR. The patient was treated with PCI as an emergency. The pattern of RBBB is new because it disappears in the subacute phase (figure b), in which an extensive anterior myocardial infarction (QS from V_1 to V_6, I, and aVL) with still present similar, but smaller ST deviations in the same leads is visible.

Which is the culprit artery of this STEMI?
a LAD proximal to D_1 and S_1
b LAD distal to D_1 and S_1
c Subocclusion of LAD involving diagonal branches

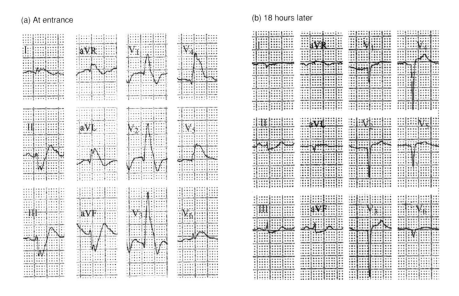

(a) At entrance

(b) 18 hours later

Answer to Case 7: a

The correct answer is **the LAD occlusion proximal to** D_1 **and** S_1.

We used the following logic:

1 A STEMI that presents on ECG with complete right branch block with ST elevation in the precordial leads, I and aVL, is due to a LAD occlusion proximal to D_1 and S_1.

2 This is because the right bundle branch is supplied by the first septal artery and because the ST elevation in I and aVL means that the occlusion is not only above the first septal artery, but also above the first diagonal artery.

3 The STEMIs with such characteristics represent a large area of risk (see Figure 12) that can cause an extensive anterior myocardial infarction as it is confirmed in (Figure b), in which the QS is seen in all precordial leads, I and aVL.

Figure 12 shows how the projection of the injury vector on the FP and HP explains the ST morphology in different leads in the case of LAD occlusion proximal to D_1 and S_1.

Pre-PCI **Post-PCI**

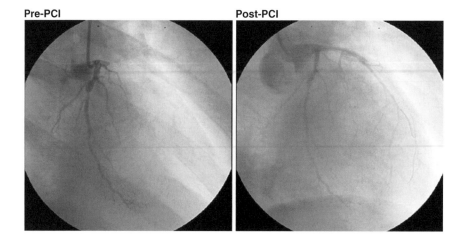

Case 8

Clinical background

A 54-year-old patient hospitalized with ischemic-type precordial pain is seen. In the first ECG (Figure a) not enough attention has been paid to the high and wide T wave in V_{1-3}, in spite of rS in V_1 and QS in V_{2-3} due to the lack of ST-segment elevation. We would like to point out that sometimes this type of T wave appears before the ST elevation. In this case, the patient remains in the hospital for further evaluation. Eighteen hours later the ECG shows a clear STEMI (Figure b) in the subacute phase, with still evident ST elevation in V_{2-4} and isoelectric ST-segment in the inferior wall leads and slightly ST elevation in V_{5-6} and depression in aVR.

Which is the culprit artery of this STEMI?

a Proximal LAD to D_1 and S_1
b Distal LAD to D_1 and S_1
c Subocclusion of LAD including the septal arteries

(a) At entrance

(b) 18 hours later

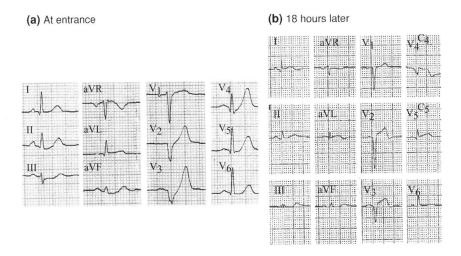

Answer to Case 8: b

The correct answer is **LAD occlusion distal to D_1 and S_1.**

We used the following logic:

1 There is no doubt that the occluded artery is LAD, because a QS pattern with ST elevation from V_2 to V_4 is present (see Figure b).

2 The presence of isoelectric ST in II, III, and aVF suggests that the occlusion is distal to D_1.

3 On the other hand, ST↑ in V_1 and aVR + ST↓ in $V_6 < 0$ suggests that the occlusion is also distal to S_1.

4 We would like to emphasize that incorrect interpretation of the first ECG (lack of appreciation that in the presence of precordial pain a wide and tall T wave in V_{1-3}, especially in the presence of QS in V_{2-3}, is very suspicious of acute ischemia) led to delay in treatment and a very bad outcome for the patient.

Figure 16 shows how the projection of the injury vector on the FP and HP explains the ST morphology in different leads in the case of LAD occlusion distal to D_1 and S_1.

Pre-PCI

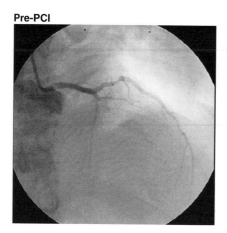

Post-PCI

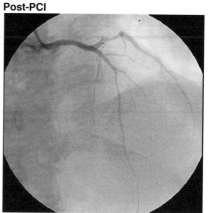

Case 9

Clinical background

A 66-year-old man presents with clinical characteristics compatible with an ACS. The ECG shows ST elevation in I and aVL with a clear ST depression in III and aVF and slight ST depression in V_{3-4}.

Which is the culprit artery of this STEMI?

a Distal LAD

b OM

c Subocclusion of LAD including diagonals or even selective occlusion of first-second diagonal (D_1–D_2)

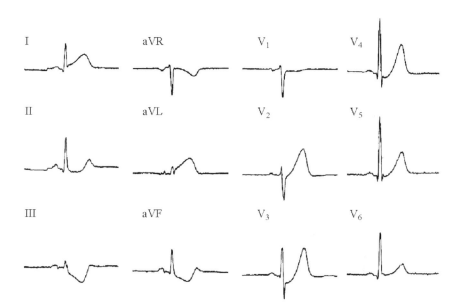

Answer to Case 9: c

The correct answer is **occlusion of D_1**.

We used the following logic:

1 There is a STEMI that especially affects I and aVL with a mirror image in III and aVF. This strongly supports the diagnosis of occlusion of the territory of the first–second diagonal arteries. In this particular case the coronary angiography demonstrates that it was a selective occlusion of D_1.

2 Often in the cases of occlusion of D_1, slight ST elevation can be seen in different precordial leads (see Figure 21). In our case there is slight ST depression in V_{2-3}. Because of this a differential diagnosis with OM occlusion has to be considered. The following data favor the D_1 occlusion:

a In the FP leads in the case of OM occlusion, ST elevation in I, aVL, and also in II, III, and aVF can be seen, or as in Case 13, ST elevation only in the inferior leads, but not ST elevation only in I and aVL, as in this case.

b Because of this, in spite of the existing ST depression in V_3 (seen more often in the cases of OM occlusion), we were convinced that in this case the occlusion is of D_1. We have observed that in the cases of occlusion of D_1 with a slight ST depression in V_{2-3}, there often exists an important stenosis of another vessel (LCX or RCA), as in this case (70% distal RCA occlusion).

c In the chronic phase, the ECG often shows QS in aVL, but not in V_{5-6}. Thus, the QS morphology in aVL usually of low voltage without Q in V_{5-6} does not correspond to a high-lateral myocardial infarction (LCX occlusion), but to a middle anterolateral myocardial infarction (D_1 occlusion) as in this case (see Figure 21).

Figure 20 shows how the projection of the injury vector on the FP and HP explains the ST morphology in different leads in the case of occlusion of the first diagonal artery.

Pre-PCI **Post-PCI**

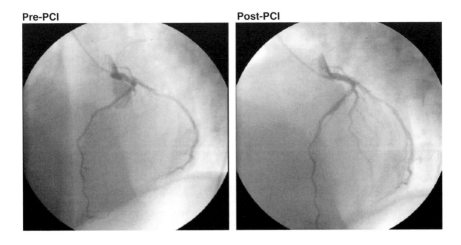

Case 10

Clinical background

A 39-year-old man presents with precordial pain that lasted for more than 24 hours and presents with some characteristics (increase with deep inspiration) that are not typical of ischemic pain. However, due to increase of the biomarkers (CPK 415, MB27, cardiac troponin I of 0.11) and diffuse ST elevation, evolving extensive anterior myocardial infarction still without Q waves was considered.

Which is the correct diagnosis?

a Proximal LAD occlusion
b Proximal RCA occlusion
c Myopericarditis

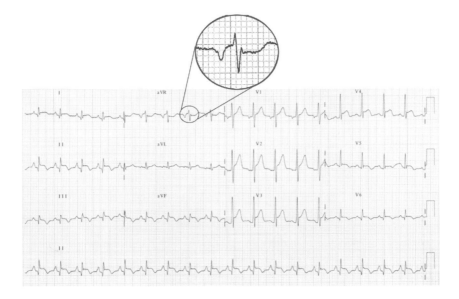

Answer to Case 10: c

The correct answer is **myopericarditis**.

We used the following logic.

The following reasons are the rationale against ACS:

1 The presence of intensive and long-standing precordial pain, but without ischemic characteristics.

2 The pain started 24 hours ago and has not generated a Q wave in spite of diffuse ST elevation.

3 Additionally, the ST elevation present in 10 leads without a mirror image and in many of them with convexity in respect to the isoelectric line (V_{1-3}) is more in favor of pericarditis than acute evolving STEMI.

4 Furthermore, the presence of evident PR elevation in aVR favors the diagnosis of pericarditis.

5 Biomarker elevation is often observed in the cases of myopericarditis. Therefore we cannot rely on this elevation to confirm myocardial infarction.

6 The coronary angiography is normal and the ECG presents a typical evolution of pericarditis (see Figure below).

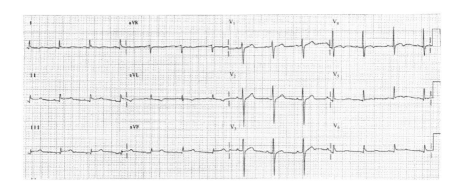

Case 11

Clinical background

A 62-year-old man presents with a visceral type thoracic pain especially in the back. The ECG shows ST elevation in the right precordial leads and ST depression in V_{5-6}, I, and aVL with very negative T wave, suggesting a "mixed pattern" (left ventricular hypertrophy and ischemia).

Because of the intense dorsal thoracic pain and the presence of an ECG with clear evidence of left ventricular hypertrophy, it was considered necessary to rule out dissecting aneurysm of the aorta.

Which is the correct diagnosis in this case?

a Proximal LAD occlusion
b Non-STEMI
c Dissecting aneurysm of the aorta

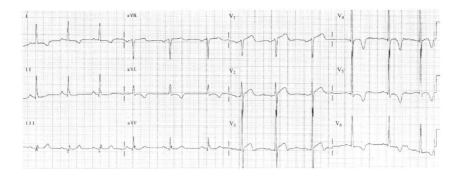

Answer to Case 11: c

The correct answer is **a dissecting aneurysm of the aorta**, which has been diagnosed using CAT scan imaging (see figure).

We used the following logic:

1 The ST elevation in V_{1-2} is a mirror image of left ventricular hypertrophy with strain, which is present in V_5 and V_6. If we look at the QRS–ST pattern elevation in V_{1-2} in detail, we realize that it is a mirror image of V_6.

2 The fact that the coronary angiography was negative and the posterior thoracic pain is present together with the characteristics of ECG makes it compulsory to rule out the presence of a dissecting aneurysm.

3 This example shows that before accepting a diagnosis for STEMI, other diseases that can cause ST elevation have to be ruled out. Some of these conditions where thoracic pain and ST elevation are present include the dissecting aneurysm, acute pericarditis, pulmonary embolism, and, in exceptional cases, pneumothorax.

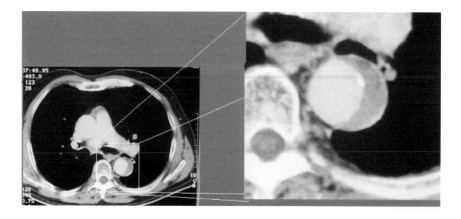

Case 12

Clinical background

A 61-year-old man was sent to our hospital for rescue PCI after being diagnosed with STEMI. Fibrinolysis was administered prior to transfer. The ECG showed ST elevation in all precordial leads, II, III, aVF (ST elevation in III is greater than that in II), and ST depression in I and aVL. There is a QR pattern in III and small rS in V_{1-3}, with sudden change to R in V_4.

Which is the culprit artery of this STEMI?

a Very proximal and very dominant RCA
b Distal occlusion of long LAD
c More than one coronary artery occlusion

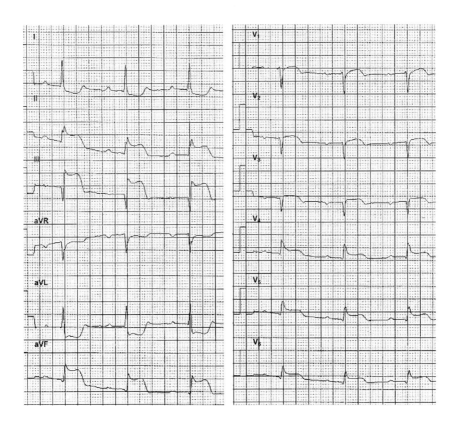

Answer to Case 12: a

The correct answer is **very proximal and very dominant RCA**.

We used the following logic.

The ECG changes can be explained by very proximal occlusion of a very dominant RCA produced by a dissecting aortic aneurysm type A affecting the RCA (see figure) instead of distal occlusion of long LAD for the following reasons (Table 2):

1 ST elevation in the inferior wall is much greater compared with ST elevation in the precordial leads, and additionally ST elevation in III is greater than that in II.

2 ST depression is very evident in I and aVL, which is not seen in the cases of distal LAD occlusion.

3 In the precordial leads V_{1-3} there is QS (small "r") with ST elevation, which can be explained by RV dilatation due to RV infarction, and in V_{4-6} there is R waves with ST elevation. ST elevation in all the precordial leads may be explained (see Table 2) by proximal involvement (ST elevation in V_{1-4}) of a very dominant (V_{4-6} ST elevation) RCA.

4 The other coronary arteries are normal.

Figure 28 shows how the projection of the injury vector on the FP and HP explains the ST morphology in different leads in the case of proximal involvement of a very dominant RCA.

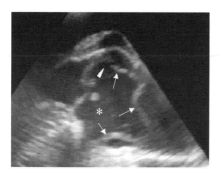 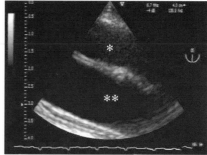

▲ Intimal tear
→ Intimal flap
* True lumen
** False lumen

Case 13

Clinical background

A 42-year-old man presents with clinical characteristics compatible with an ACS without hemodynamic compromise.

The ECG shows:

1 Slight ST elevation in II, III, and aVF
2 ST depression in V_{1-3} with isodiphasic ST in lead I

Which is the culprit artery of this STEMI?

a Nondominant RCA
b Proximal LCX
c Obtuse marginal

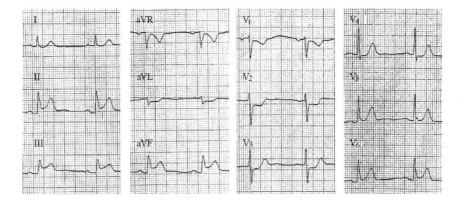

Answer to Case 13: c

The correct answer is **obtuse marginal**.

In this case the logic we used did not lead us to a definitive conclusion. ST in I is isodiphasic, ST elevation in III is very similar to that in II, and finally the ratio ST depression in V_{1-3}/ST elevation in II, III, VF is around 1. The relatively small deviations of ST favor distal occlusion of RCA or LCX, including OM occlusion. The coronary angiography demonstrated that the occlusion was of a large OM.

However, in general, in the case of OM occlusion the ST elevation is present not only in the inferior leads, but also in the lateral leads, since the injury vector is more frequently directed approximately towards $0°$ (see Figures 32 and 33). In this case, on the contrary, it is positioned between $+60°$ and $+90°$ (negative in aVL and isoelectric in I).

This case demonstrates that occasionally, especially when the changes of ST are not striking, it is difficult to localize the injury vector and additionally, the anatomic variation from patient to patient makes it difficult to identify through the ST changes the precise culprit coronary artery supplying this particular region of the inferolateral zone of the heart. In our experience this happens in less than 10–15% of cases.

Figure 32 shows how the projection of the injury vector on the FP and HP explains the most typical ST morphology in different leads in the case of obtuse marginal occlusion.

Pre-PCI

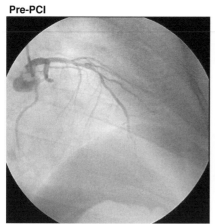

Post-PCI

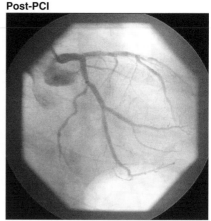

Case 14

Clinical background

A 46-year-old man presents with acute ischemic type chest pain of 8 hours' duration.

The ECG shows:

1 ST elevation in II, III, aVF, and V_{5-6}
2 ST depression in I, aVL, V_1, and V_2
3 Q waves in III and VF

Which is the culprit artery of this STEMI?

a RCA proximal
b RCA distal and dominant
c LCX proximal

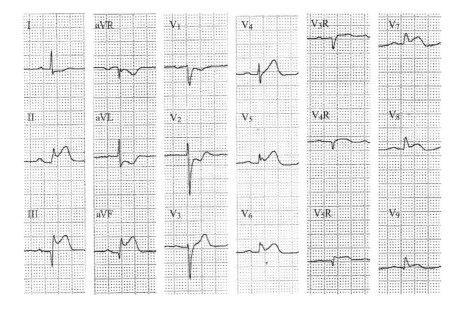

Answer to Case 14: b

The correct answer is **dominant RCA with distal occlusion**.

We used the following logic:

1 The culprit artery is the RCA. According to the algorithm presented in Figure 37, this case illustrates the following:

a ST depression in I

b ST elevation in III greater than that in II

c $\sum ST\downarrow$ in $V_{1-3}/\sum ST\uparrow$ in II, III, VF < 1

4 RCA occlusion is probably distal because there is ST segment depression in V_{1-2}. In this case lead V_4R favors proximal occlusion. The coronary angiography demonstrates that the occlusion was distal.

5 RCA is dominant because there is ST elevation in V_{5-6} but not very dominant because in these leads the ST$\uparrow$ < 2 mm.

Figure 28 shows how the projection of the injury vector on the FP and HP explains the ST morphology in different leads in the case of a dominant RCA with distal occlusion.

Pre-PCI

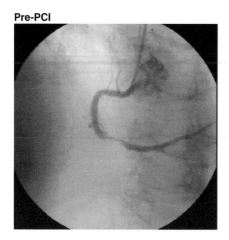

Post-PCI

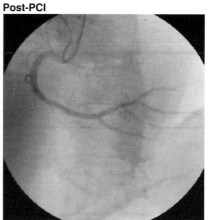

Case 15

Clinical background

A 54-year-old man presents with acute precordial pain and clinical characteristics compatible with an ACS.

The ECG shows:

1 ST depression from V_1 to V_{3-4} as the most striking alterations
2 ST elevation not so evident in II, III, aVF and a bit more evident in V_6
3 Slight ST depression in aVL and even smaller in I

Which is the culprit artery of this ACS?

a STEMI due to very dominant RCA
b STEMI due to very dominant LCX
c Non-STEMI due to LAD coronary artery subocclusion

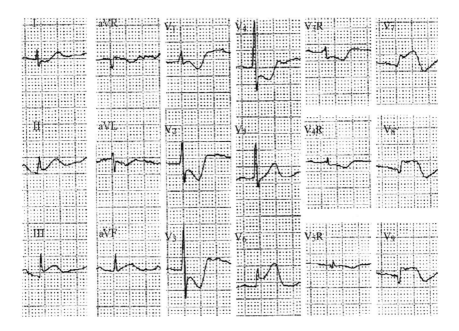

Answer to Case 15: b

The correct answer is a **very dominant LCX** (see coronary angiography).

We used the following logic:

1 Even though we observe ST depression in V_{1-4} as the most striking alteration, this case is not a NSTEMI, because although not striking, there is ST elevation in the inferior leads and V_6. It is known that, with certain frequency, in the cases of STEMI due to occlusion of the LCX, and especially when the inferobasal segment of the inferior wall is truly posterior (see p. 39), the ST depression in the precordial leads V_{1-4} is sometimes much more evident than the ST elevation in the inferior leads.

2 The ST depression in the precordial leads V_{1-4} cannot be due to LAD occlusion. If this were the case, there would not be elevation either in V_6 or in the inferior leads.

3 The LCX has to be very dominant to show ST depression in aVL even though it is not so evident in I. In our experience the only cases of ST elevation in II, III, and aVF that present with ST depression in lead I and that are not due to RCA occlusion are the result of a very dominant LCX occlusion. In the cases of very dominant RCA, ST elevation in II, III, and aVF would be much more evident compared with ST depression in V_{1-4}, and the depression in I and especially in aVL would be much more striking than in this case of LCX occlusion.

4 In this case extreme right precordial and posterior leads have been recorded. The extreme right precordial leads show ST depression with a negative T wave, which points toward occlusion of the LCX (Figure 37) and the posterior leads give us a mirror image of V_{1-3}. Even though the assessment of these leads is not completely necessary for the correct diagnosis, the pattern observed in V_3–V_4R also strongly supports the occlusion of LCX.

5 The case of Figure 35, which also corresponds to the occlusion of very dominant LCX, presents complete occlusion of LCX (compare coronarographies of two cases) and consequently a bigger burden of ischemia. The sum of ST deviations in the case of Figure 35 is much higher than in this case where the occlusion of LCX is not complete (48 mm vs 22 mm). We reiterate that the prognosis is very poor when the sum of ST deviations is greater than 15 mm.

Figure 34 shows how the projection of the injury vector on the FP and HP explains the ST morphology in different leads in the case of a very dominant LCX.

Pre-PCI   Post-PCI

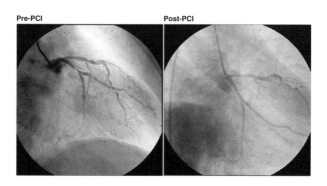

References

Bayés de Luna A. Textbook of Clinical Electrocardiography. New York: Futura Publishing; 1999.

Bayes de Luna A, Fiol M. El ECG de la cardiopatía isquémica: correlaciones clínicas y de imagen e implicaciones pronósticas. Barcelona Prous Science; 2006.

Bayés de Luna A, Malik M. Electrocardiography. In: Camm J, Serruys P, Luscher J, eds. Textbook of Cardiology. London: Blackwell Publishers; 2005.

Birnbaum Y, Hasdai D, Sclarovsky S, Herz I, Strasberg B, Rechavia E. Acute myocardial infarction entailing ST segment elevation in lead AVL: electrocardiographic differentiation among occlusion of the left anterior descending, first diagonal and first obtuse marginal coronary arteries. Am Heart J 1996;131:38.

Birnbaum Y, Sclarovsky S, Blum A, Mager A, Gabbay U. Prognostic significance of the initial electrocardiographic pattern in a first acute anterior wall myocardial infarction. Chest 1993;103:1681.

Birnbaum Y, Solodky A, Herz I, et al. Implications of inferior ST-segment depression in anterior acute myocardial infarction: electrocardiographic and angiographic correlation. Am Heart J 1994;127:1467.

Blackwell GB, Cranney GB, Pohost GM. Slide Atlas of MRI: Cardiovascular System. London: Gower Medical Publishing; 1993.

Chou Te-Chuan, Helm RA, Kaplan S. Clinical Vectocardiography. New York: Grune & Stratton;1977.

Engelen DJ, Gorgels AP, Cheriex EC, et al. Value of the electrocardiogram in localizing the occlusion site in the left anterior descending coronary artery in acute anterior myocardial infarction. J Am Coll Cardiol 1999;34:389.

Eskola M, Nikus K, Niemelä K, Sclarovsky S. How to use ECG for decision support in the catheterization laboratory. Cases with inferior ST segment elevaton acute coronary syndrome. J Electrocardiol 2004;37:257.

Finn A, Antman E. Images in clinical medicine: isolated right ventricular infarction. N Engl J Med 2003;349:17.

Fiol M, Carrillo A, Cygankiewicz I, et al. New criteria based on ST changes in 12 leads surface ECG to detect proximal vs distal right coronary artery occlusion in case of an acute inferoposterior myocardial infarction. Ann Noninvasive Electrocardiol 2004a;9(4):383.

Fiol M, Cino J, Cygankiewicz I, et al. The value of an algorithm based on ST segment deviations to locate the place of occlussion in left anterior descending coronary artery in case of ST-segment elevation-myocardial infarction. 2006. (Submitted)

Fiol M, Cygankiewicz I, Guindo J, et al. Evolving myocardial infarction with ST elevation: ups and downs of ST in different leads identifies the culprit artery and location of the occlusion. Ann Noninvasive Electrocardiol 2004b;9:180.

Fiol M, Cygankiewicz I, Carillo A, et al. Value of electrocardiographic algorithm based on 'Ups and Downs' of ST in assessment of a culprit artery in evolving inferior myocardial infarction. Am J Cardiol 2004c;94:709.

Fiol M, Marrugat J, Bayés de Luna A, Bergada J, Guindo J. Ventricular fibrillation markers on admission to the hospital for acute myocardial infarction. Am J Cardiol 1993;71: 117.

Gallik DM, Obermueller SD, Swarna US, Guidry GW, Mahmarian JJ, Verani MS. Simultaneous assessment of myocardial perfusion and left ventricular dysfunction during transient coronary occlusion. J Am Coll Cardiol 1995;25:1529.

Goldman M.J. Principles of Clinical Electrocardiography. San Francisco: LPM Publishers;1964.

Haraphongse M, Tanomsup S, Jugdutt BI. Inferior ST segment depression during acute anterior myocardial infarction: clinical and angiographic correlations. J Am Coll Cardiol 1984;4:467.

Hathaway WR, Peterson ED, Wagner GS, et al, for the GUSTO-I Investigators. Prognostic significance of the initial electrocardiogram in patients with acute myocardial infarction. JAMA 1998;279:387.

Herz I, Assali AR, Adler Y, Solodky A, Sclarovsky S. New electrocardiographic criteria for predicting either the right or left circumflex artery as the culprit coronary artery in inferior wall acute myocardial infarction. Am J Cardiol 1997;80:1343.

Karmpaliotis D, Turakhia MP, Kirtane AJ, et al. Sequential risk stratification using TIMI risk score and TIMI flow grade among patients treated with fibrinolytic therapy for ST-segment elevation acute myocardial infarction. Am J Cardiol Nov 1, 2004;94(9):1113.

Kennedy RJ, Varriale P, Alfenito JC.Texbook of Vectocardiography. New Jersey: Harper and Row; 1970.

Kosuge M, Kimura K, Ishikawa T, et al. New electrocardiographic criteria for predicting the site of coronary artery occlusion in inferior wall acute myocardial infarction. Am J Cardiol 1998;82:1318.

Kosuge M, Kimura K, Ishikawa T, Toshiak E, Setoshi V. Predictors of left-main or three vessel disease in patients who have acute coronary syndromes with non-ST segment elevation. Am J Cardiol 2005;95:1366.

Kurum T, Oztekin E, Ozcelik F, Eker H, Ture M, Ozbay G. Predictive value of admission electrocardiogram for multivessel disease in acute anterior and anterior-inferior myocardial infarction. Ann Noninvasive Electrocardiol 2002;7:369.

Leibrand PN, Bell SJ, Savona MR, et al. Validation of cardiologist's decisions to initiate reperfusion therapy with ECG viewed on liquid crystal displays of cellular phones. Am Heart J 2000;140:747.

Lew AS, Laramee P, Shah PK, Maddahi J, Peter T, Ganz W. Ratio of ST-segment depression in lead V2 to ST-segment elevation in lead aVF in evolving inferior acute myocardial infarction: an aid to the early recognition of right ventricular ischemia. Am J Cardiol 1986; 57:1047.

Martinez-Dolz L, Arnau MA, Almenar L, et al. Utilidad del ECG en la predicción del lugar de la oclusión en el infarto agudo de miocardio en el síndrome coronario agudo debido a oclusión de la arteria descendente anterior aislada. Rev Esp Cardiol 2002;55(10): 1036.

Nikus KC, Eskola MJ, Virtanem VK, et al. ST depression with negative T waves in leads V4-5 – a marker of severe coronary artery disease in non-ST elevation acute coronary syndromes. Ann Noninvasive Electrocardiol 2004;9:207.

Nikus C, Sclarovsky S, Eskola M, Niemelä K. Modern morphologic electrocardiographic interpretation – a valuable tool for rapid clinical decision making in acute ishemic coronary syndromes [editorial comment]. J Electrocardiol 2005;38:4.

Pons-Lladó G, Carreras F. Atlas of Practical Applications of Cardiovascular Magnetic Resonance. New York: Springer; 2005.

Porter A, Sclarovsky S, Ben-Gal T, Herz I, Solodky A, Sagie A. Value of T-wave direction with lead III ST-segment depression in acute anterior wall myocardial infarction: electrocardiographic prediction of a 'wrapped' left anterior descending artery. Clin Cardiol 1998;21:562.

Prieto JA, González C, Hernández MA, De la Torre JM, Llorca J. Predicción electrocardiográfica de la localización de la lesión en la arteria descendente anterior en el infarto agudo de miocardio. Rev Esp Cardiol 2002;55:1028.

Roberts WC, Gardin JM. Location of myocardial infarcts: a confusion of terms and definitions. Am J Cardiol 1978;42:868.

Sadananden S, Hochman S, Kolodzjez A, et al. Clnical and angiographic characteristics of patients with combined anterior and inferior ST segment elevation in the initial electrocardiogram during acute myocardial infarction. Am Heart J 2003;146:653.

Sapin P, Musselman DR, Dehmer GJ, Cascio WE. Implications of inferior ST-segment elevation accompanying anterior wall acute myocardial infarction for the angiographic morphology of the left anterior descending coronary artery morphology and site of occlusion. Am J Cardiol 1992;69:860.

Saw J, DaviesC, Fung A, Spinelli JJ, Jue J. Value of ST elevation in lead III greater than lead II in inferior wall acute myocardial infarction for predicting in-hospital mortality and diagnosing right ventricular infarction. Am J Cardiol 2001;87:448.

Schmitt C, Günter L, Scmieder S, Karch M, Neuman FJ, Schömig A. Diagnosis of acute myocardial infarction in angiographically documented occluded infarct vessel. Limitations of ST elevation in standard and extended ECG leads. Chest 2001;120:1540.

Sclarowsky, S. Electrocardiography of Acute Myocardial Ischemia. London: Martin Dunitz;1999.

Tamura A, Kataoka H, Mikuriya Y, Nasu M. Inferior ST segment depression as a useful marker for identifying proximal left anterior descending artery occlusion during acute anterior myocardial infarction. Eur Heart J 1995;16:1795.

Tamura A, Kataoka H, Mikuriya Y. Electrocardiographic findings in a patient with pure septal infarction. Br Heart J Mar 1991;65(3):166.

Wagner GS. Marriot's Electrocardiography. Philadelphia: Williams and Wilkins; 2002.

Wellens HJ, Gorgels A, Doevendans PA. The ECG in acute myocardial infarction and unstable angina. Boston: Kluwer Academic Publishers, 2003.

Yamaji H, Iwasaki K, Kusachi S, et al. Prediction of acute left main coronary artery obstruction by 12-lead electrocardiography. ST segment elevation in lead a VR with less ST segment elevation in lead V1. J Am Coll Cardiol 2001;38:1348.

Zalenski RJ, Rydman RJ, Sloan EP, et al. Value of posterior and right ventricular leads in comparison to the standard 12-lead electrocardiogram in evaluation of ST-segment elevation in suspected acute myocardial infarction. Am J Cardiol 1997;79:1579.

Index

Note: page numbers in **bold** refer to tables, those in *italics* refer to figures